GERIATRICS *At Your* FINGERTIPS

2002 EDITION

GERIATRICS *At Your* FINGERTIPS

2002 EDITION

AUTHORS:

David B. Reuben, MD

Keela A. Herr, PhD, RN

James T. Pacala, MD, MS

Jane F. Potter, MD

Bruce G. Pollock, MD, PhD

Todd P. Semla, MS, PharmD

PUBLISHED BY BLACKWELL SCIENCE, INC.
MALDEN, MA, USA

This publication was prepared by Blackwell Science, Inc., at the direction of the American Geriatrics Society as a service to health care providers involved in the care of older persons. Funding for the first edition of this book provided by the John A. Hartford Foundation made the development of this publication possible.

Although *Geriatrics At Your Fingertips* is distributed by various companies in the health care field, it is independently prepared and published. All decisions regarding its content are solely the responsibility of the authors. Their decisions are not subject to any form of approval by other interests or organizations.

Some recommendations in this publication suggest the use of agents for purposes or in dosages other than those recommended in product labeling. Such recommendations are based on reports in peer-reviewed publications and are not based on or influenced by any material or advice from pharmaceutical or health care product manufacturers.

No responsibility is assumed by the authors or the American Geriatrics Society for any injury or damage to persons or property, as a matter of product liability, negligence, warranty, or otherwise, arising out of the use or application of any methods, products, instructions, or ideas contained herein. No guarantee, endorsement, or warranty of any kind, express or implied (including specifically no warrant of merchantability or of fitness for a particular purpose) is given by the Society in connection with any information contained herein. Independent verification of any diagnosis, treatment, or drug use or dosage should be obtained. No test or procedure should be performed unless, in the judgment of an independent, qualified physician, it is justified in the light of the risk involved.

Citation: Reuben DB, Herr K, Pacala JT, *et al. Geriatrics At Your Fingertips: 2002 Edition.* Malden, MA: Blackwell Science, Inc., for the American Geriatrics Society; 2002.

ISBN 0-632-04696-1
Library of Congress Catalog Card Number 2001008152
Printed in the U.S.A.

TABLE OF CONTENTS

AUTHORS

David B. Reuben, MD
Director, Multicampus Program in Geriatric Medicine and Gerontology
Chief, Division of Geriatrics
Professor of Medicine
UCLA School of Medicine
Los Angeles, CA

Keela A. Herr, PhD, RN
Professor
College of Nursing
The University of Iowa
Iowa City, IA

James T. Pacala, MD, MS
Associate Professor and Vice Chair for Medical Student Affairs
Department of Family Practice and Community Health
University of Minnesota
Minneapolis, MN

Bruce G. Pollock, MD, PhD
Professor of Psychiatry, Pharmacology, and Pharmaceutical Sciences
Chief, Academic Division of Geriatrics and Neuropsychiatry
Department of Psychiatry, University of Pittsburgh
Pittsburgh, PA

Jane F. Potter, MD
Chief, Section of Geriatrics and Gerontology
Harris Professor of Geriatric Medicine
University of Nebraska Medical Center
Omaha, NE

Todd P. Semla, MS, PharmD
Department of Psychiatry and Behavioral Sciences
Evanston Northwestern Healthcare
Evanston, IL
Clinical Assistant Professor
Section of Geriatric Medicine
College of Medicine
University of Illinois at Chicago
Chicago, IL

ABBREVIATIONS

ABG	arterial blood gas
ac	before meals (*ante cibum*)
ACC	American College of Cardiology
ACE	angiotensin-converting enzyme
ACIP	Advisory Committee on Immunization Practices
ACOG	American College of Obstetrics and Gynecology
ACR	American College of Rheumatology
AD	Alzheimer's disease
ADA	American Diabetes Association
ADLs	activities of daily living
AFB	acid-fast bacillus
AHA	American Heart Association
AHCPR	Agency for Health Care Policy and Research
	(now, Agency for Healthcare Research and Quality)
AIDS	acquired immune deficiency syndrome
AIMS	Abnormal Involuntary Movement Scale
ALT	alanine aminotransferase
ASA	American Society of Anesthesiologists
ATA	American Thyroid Association
ATS	American Thoracic Society
AUA	American Urological Association
bid	twice a day (*bis in die*)
BIPAP	bilevel positive airway pressure
BMD	bone mineral density
BMI	body mass index
BP	blood pressure
BPH	benign prostatic hyperplasia
BUN	blood urea nitrogen
C&S	culture and sensitivity
CABG	coronary artery bypass graft
CAD	coronary artery disease
CAPD	central auditory processing disorder
CBC	complete blood cell count
CBT	cognitive behavior therapy
cfu	colony-forming unit
CHD	coronary heart disease
CHF	congestive heart failure
CI	confidence interval
CNS	central nervous system
COPD	chronic obstructive pulmonary disease
CPAP	continuous positive airway pressure
CPK	creatine phosphokinase
CPR	cardiopulmonary resuscitation

Cr	creatinine
CrCl	creatinine clearance
CT	*chewable tablet or* computed tomography
CXR	chest x-ray
CYP	cytochrome P-450
d	day(s)
D&C	dilation and curettage
D5W	dextrose 5% in water
DBP	diastolic blood pressure
D/C	discontinue
DHIC	detrusor hyperactivity with impaired contractility
DSM-IV	*Diagnostic and Statistical Manual of Mental Disorders*, 4th ed. (Washington, DC: American Psychiatric Association; 1994)
DTR	deep-tendon reflex
DVT	deep-vein thrombosis
ECF	extracellular fluid
ECG	electrocardiogram, electrocardiography
EF	ejection fraction
EPS	extrapyramidal symptoms
ESR	erythrocyte sedimentation rate
F	feces, fecal (elimination, in drug tables)
FDA	Food and Drug Administration
FEV_1	forced expiratory volume in 1 second
FOBT	fecal occult blood test
FVC	forced vital capacity
GAD	generalized anxiety disorder
GDS	Geriatric Depression Scale
GERD	gastroesophageal reflux disease
GFR	glomerular filtration rate
GI	gastrointestinal
GU	genitourinary
h	hour(s)
Hb	hemoglobin
HbA_{1c}	glycosylated hemoglobin
HDL	high-density lipoprotein
HR	heart rate
HRT	hormone replacement therapy
hs	at bedtime (*hora somni*)
HTN	hypertension
hx	history
IADLs	instrumental activities of daily living
IBW	ideal body weight
IM	intramuscular(ly)
INH	isoniazid
INR	international normalized ratio
IOP	intraocular pressure
IPC	intermittent pneumatic compression
IT	intrathecal

IV	intravenous(ly)
JNC-VI	Sixth Joint National Committee on Prevention, Detection, Evaluation, and Treatment of High Blood Pressure
K	kidney (metabolism and excretion, in drug tables)
K+	potassium ion
L	liver (metabolism and excretion, in drug tables)
LBW	lean body weight
LDL	low-density lipoprotein
LDUH	low-dose unfractionated heparin
LFT	liver function test
LMWH	low-molecular-weight heparin
LVH	left ventricular hypertrophy
MAOI	monoamine oxidase inhibitor
MDI	metered-dose inhaler
MI	myocardial infarction
min	minute(s)
MMSE	Folstein's Mini–Mental State Examination
MSE	mental status examination
mo	month(s)
MRI	magnetic resonance imaging
NG	nasogastric
NS	normal saline
NSAIDs	nonsteroidal anti-inflammatory drugs
NPH	neutral protamine Hagedorn (insulin)
npo	nothing by mouth (*non per os*)
OCD	obsessive-compulsive disorder
OGTT	oral glucose tolerance test
OT	occupational therapy
OTC	over-the-counter
pc	after a meal (*post cibum*)
PE	pulmonary embolism
PEF	peak expiratory flow
PET	positron emission tomography
PNS	peripheral nervous system
po	by mouth (*per os*)
POMA	Performance-Oriented Mobility Assessment
PPD	purified protein derivative (of tuberculin)
prn	as needed (*pro re nata*)
PSA	prostate-specific antigen
PT	prothrombin time *or* physical therapy
PTCA	percutaneous transluminal coronary angioplasty
PTT	partial thromboplastin time
PUVA	psoralen plus ultraviolet light of A wavelength
qam	every morning (*quaque ante meridiem*)
qd	every day (*quaque die*)
qhs	each bedtime (*quaque hora somni*)
qid	four times a day (*quater in die*)
qod	every other day (*quaque altera die*)

QT$_c$	QT (cardiac output) corrected for heart rate
RBC	ranitidine bismuth citrate *or* red blood cells
sats	saturations
SD	standard deviation
SBP	systolic blood pressure
SC	subcutaneous(ly)
sec	second(s)
SIADH	syndrome of inappropriate secretion of antidiuretic hormone
sl	according to rules (*secundum legem*)
SOB	shortness of breath
SPECT	single-photon emission computed tomography
SPEP	serum protein electrophoresis
SR	sustained release
SSRIs	selective serotonin-reuptake inhibitors
TCA	tricyclic antidepressant
TD	tardive dyskinesia
TDD	telephone device for the deaf
TG	triglycerides
TIA	transient ischemic attack
tid	three times a day (*ter in die*)
TSG	thyroid-stimulating globulin
TSH	thyroid-stimulating hormone
TTP	thrombotic thrombocytopenic purpura
TUIP	transurethral incision of the prostate
TURP	transurethral resection of the prostate
U	unit(s)
UA	urinalysis
UI	urinary incontinence
UV	ultraviolet
VIN	vulvar intraepithelial neoplasia
WHO	World Health Organization
wk	week(s)
wt	weight
yr	year(s)

Drug Tables

Drug trade names are in *italic* type. **Bold** type indicates preferred drugs for treating older persons. Drug formulations are in brackets and expressed in mg (milligrams) unless specified otherwise, and the following abbreviations indicate forms:
C = capsule; CR = controlled release; CT = chewable tablet; ER = extended release; Inj = injectable; S = liquid; Sp = suppository; SR = sustained release; T = tablet; TR = timed release.

INTRODUCTION

To provide high-quality medical care for older persons requires a special set of knowledge, clinical skills, and attitudes. Many resources that provide current, accurate information on patient evaluation and management are available. However, few of these are portable enough to be used in the examining room, on nursing home or hospital rounds, or when the clinician is on call outside the office.

In 1998, the American Geriatrics Society (AGS) first published *Geriatrics At Your Fingertips*, a pocket guide that provided immediate access to specific information needed to care for older persons in various health care settings. The response to the first three editions was extraordinary, and *Geriatrics At Your Fingertips* soon became the society's best-selling publication. In preparing this fourth edition, we have tried to incorporate suggestions about format and content from readers of prior editions. Specifically, we have combined the drug and subject indexes into one index. We have added content (eg, information on aortic valve disease and a guide to important cytochrome P-450 drug interactions), and we have updated information throughout the text and tables.

Like its predecessors, this new guide provides assessment instruments, recommended diagnostic tests, and management strategies, including nonpharmacologic and pharmacologic therapy. Tables and lists of drugs are designed to facilitate appropriate prescribing. Generic and trade names are provided, as well as information on dosages, how the drugs are metabolized or excreted, and how each drug is supplied. Frequently, the duration of action and specific cautions to be observed when using the medication in older persons are also supplied.

The goal of *Geriatrics at Your Fingertips* is to reduce to a minimum the amount of time that a practicing clinician must spend searching for specific information that is needed immediately to make patient care decisions. Accordingly, the book does not attempt to explain in detail the rationale underlying the strategies presented. In many instances, these strategies have been derived from guidelines published by organizations such as the Agency for Healthcare Research and Quality, the American Heart Association, and the American Diabetes Association. Many of the guidelines can be obtained from the National Guidelines Clearinghouse (www.guideline.gov). When no such guidelines exist, the strategies recommended herein represent the best opinions of the authors and the experts they have asked to review the chapters. In an effort to be comprehensive yet concise, references have been provided sparingly, but many others that are relevant are available from the organizations mentioned or in the most recent edition of the AGS *Geriatrics Review Syllabus*.

The authors welcome comments about the format and content of this edition of *Geriatrics At Your Fingertips* that may guide the preparation of future editions. All comments should be addressed to the American Geriatrics Society, Empire State Building, 350 Fifth Avenue, Suite 801, New York, NY 10118.

The authors are particularly grateful to Nancy Lundebjerg at the AGS, who has served a vital role in the development of this book and its readership. We are also grateful to the John A. Hartford Foundation for support in distributing *Geriatrics At Your Fingertips* to medical students and residents across the nation.

We would also like to thank the following persons who have reviewed portions of the text that lie within their expertise:

Wendy L. Adams, MD

David McCulloch, MD

Victoria Braund, MD

Alison Moore, MD

Catherine Dubeau, MD

Patricia Morrow, MS

Bruce A. Ferrell, MD

Benoit H. Mulsant, MD

John FitzGerald, MD

Lauren Nathan, MD

Rita A. Frantz, PhD, RN

Joseph Ouslander, MD

Gail Greendale, MD

John Song, MD

Thomas Hejkel, MD

Mary Tinetti, MD

Alan Hirsh, MD

Cynthia Toher, MD

Margaret A. Kessinger, MD

James Webster, MD

Saman Lashkari, MD

Thomas T. Yoshikawa, MD

The following organizations have issued guidelines that have been the basis of parts of specific chapters:

Advisory Committee on Immunization Practices
Agency for Health Care Policy and Research
   (now, Agency for Healthcare Research and Quality)
Alzheimer's Association
Amercian Academy of Neurology
American Association for Geriatric Psychiatry
American College of Cardiology
American College of Chest Physicians
American College of Gastroenterology
American College of Obstetrics and Gynecology
American College of Rheumatology
American Diabetes Association
American Geriatrics Society
American Heart Association
American Lung Association
American Pain Society
American Psychiatric Association
American Society of Anesthesiologists
American Thoracic Society
American Thyroid Association
American Urological Association
National Cholesterol Education Program
National Heart, Lung, and Blood Institute
U.S. Preventive Services Task Force
World Health Organization

The following persons have assisted the authors in planning and assembling the 2002 edition:

Managing Editor: Carol S. Goodwin
Medical Editor: Barbara B. Reitt, PhD, ELS(D), Reitt Editing Services
Medical Indexer: L. Pilar Wyman, Wyman Indexing

READY REFERENCE

AGE-RELATED PHYSIOLOGIC CHANGES AND FORMULAS

Table 1. Conversions		
Temperature	**Liquid**	**Weight**
F = (1.8)C + 32	1 fl dram = 4 mL	1 lb = 0.453 kg
C = (F − 32) / (1.8)	1 fl oz = 30 mL	1 kg = 2.2 lb
	1 tsp = 5 mL	1 oz = 30 g
	1 tbsp = 15 mL	1 grain = 60 mg

FORMULAS

Alveolar-Arterial Oxygen Gradient $A - a = 148 - 1.2(Paco_2) - Pao_2$
[normal = 10 − 20 mm Hg, breathing room air at sea level]

Calculated Osmolality
2Na + glucose / 18 + BUN / 2.8 + ethanol / 4.6 + isopropanol / 6 + methanol / 3.2 + ethylene glycol / 6.2   [normal = 280 − 295]

Golden Rules of Arterial Blood Gases
• Pco_2 change of 10 corresponds to a pH change of 0.08.
• pH change of 0.15 corresponds to base excess change of 10 mEq/L.

Creatinine Clearance
For renally eliminated drugs, dosage adjustments may be necessary if CrCl < 60.

$$\frac{IBW(140 - age)(0.85 \text{ if female})}{(72)(\text{stable creatinine})}$$

Erythrocyte Sedimentation Rate
Westergren: women = (age + 10) / 2
            men = age / 2

Ideal Body Weight
• Male = 50 kg + (2.3 kg)(each inch of height > 5 feet)
• Female = 45.5 kg + (2.3 kg)(each inch of height > 5 feet)

Lean Body Weight
IBW + 0.4 (actual body weight − IBW)

Body Mass Index

$$\frac{\text{weight in kg}}{(\text{height in meters})^2} \quad or \quad \frac{\text{weight in lb}}{(\text{height in inches})^2} \times 704.5$$

Partial Pressure of Oxygen, Arterial (Pao_2) While Breathing Room Air
100 − (age/3) estimates decline

Table 2. Motor Function by Nerve Roots			
Level	**Motor Function**	**Level**	**Motor Function**
C4	Spontaneous breathing	L1–L2	Hip flexion
C5	Shoulder shrug	L3	Hip adduction
C6	Elbow flexion	L4	Hip abduction
C7	Elbow extension	L5	Great toe dorsiflexion
C8/T1	Finger flexion	S1–S2	Foot plantar flexion
T1–T12	Intercostal abdominal muscles	S2–S4	Rectal tone

Table 3. Lumbosacral Nerve Root Compression			
Root	**Motor**	**Sensory**	**Reflex**
L4	Quadriceps	Medial foot	Knee-jerk
L5	Dorsiflexors	Dorsum of foot	Medial hamstring
S1	Plantar flexors	Lateral foot	Ankle-jerk

Figure 1. Dermatomes

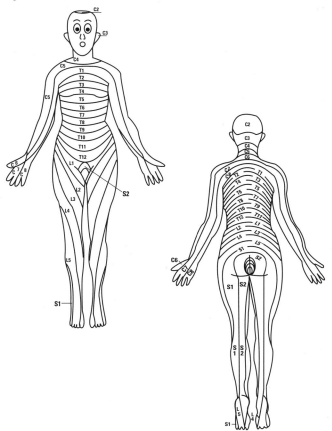

Source: *The 1999 Tarascon Pocket Pharmacopoeia.* Loma Linda, CA: Tarascon Publishing Company; 1999:7.
Reprinted with permission.

3

ASSESSMENT AND APPROACH

ASSESSMENT

Table 4. Dimensions of Assessment*		
Domain, Dimension	**Method**	**See Page**
Medical		
Medical status	Hx, physical examination, laboratory tests	4
Medications	Medications review	8–11
Nutrition	Dietary hx	84
Dentition	Dental examination	
Mental, emotional		
Cognitive status	Mental status examination, eg, Mini-Cog, MMSE	161
Emotional status	Depression screen, eg, GDS	165
Physical function		
Functional status	ADLs, IADLs	163, 164
Balance and gait	Physical evaluation, POMA scale	167
Environmental		
Social, financial status	Social hx	
Environmental hazards	Home evaluation	58

Note: For information on clinical uses of the domain management model, see Siebens H. Applying the domain management model in treating patients with chronic diseases. *J Qual Improvement* 2001;27(6):302–314.
* See Assessment Instruments, pp 161–173.

Review of Systems
Make sure to inquire about:
- Bowel patterns, especially constipation
- Cardiovascular system (eg, chest pain, SOB, claudication)
- Dizziness
- Falls
- Fatigue
- Functional change over past year or since last visit
- Hearing (see p 166) or visual changes
- Medication use (see p 8)
- Musculoskeletal stiffness or pain
- Sleep patterns
- Urinary patterns, especially incontinence
- Weight change

Physical Examination
Make sure to check:
- Height and weight
- Orthostatic BP, pulse
- Skin integrity (all surfaces)
- Vision and hearing

NURSING-HOME ASSESSMENT
Admissions Checklist
1. History, physical, labs as needed; PPD
2. Determine functional status: ADL, IADL, MSE, depression scale
3. Review medications (correlate to active diagnoses)
4. Identify medical conditions—review old records

5. Assess for presence of pain
6. Establish relationships—resident, family, staff
7. Establish advance directives
8. Formulate problem list
9. Formulate plan

Scheduled Visit Checklist
1. Evaluate patient for interval functional change
2. Check vital signs, weight, labs, consultant reports since last visit
3. Review medications (correlate to active diagnoses)
4. Sign orders
5. Address nursing staff concerns
6. Write a SOAP note (subjective data, objective data, assessment, plan)
7. Revise problem list as needed
8. Update advance directives at least yearly
9. Update resident; update family member(s) as needed

Health Maintenance
Yearly: Functional status, MSE, depression screen, vision, hearing, dental, podiatric, history, physical, creatinine, hemoglobin, TSH in women; other labs and preventive procedures to be decided individually
Monthly: Weight, vital signs
Ongoing: Skin integrity, pain assessment
Immunizations: influenza vaccine once/yr in the fall months; pneumococcal vaccine (*Pneumovax 23, Pnu-Immune 23*) once at age 65; consider repeat every 6–7 yr; tetanus vaccine every 10 yr

INFORMED DECISION MAKING (see **Figure 2**)
Three elements are needed for a patient's choices to be legally, ethically valid:
• A capable decision maker: Capacity is to the decision being made; patient may be capable of making some but not all decisions. For a sufficiently impaired person, a surrogate decision maker must be involved.
• Patient's voluntary participation in the decision-making process.
• Sufficient information: Patient must be sufficiently informed; items to disclose in informed consent include:
  - Diagnosis
  - Nature, risks, costs, and benefits of possible interventions
  - Alternative treatments; relative benefits, risks, and costs
  - Likely results of no treatment
  - Likelihood of success
  - Advice or recommendation of the clinician

Figure 2. Algorithm for Informed Decision Making

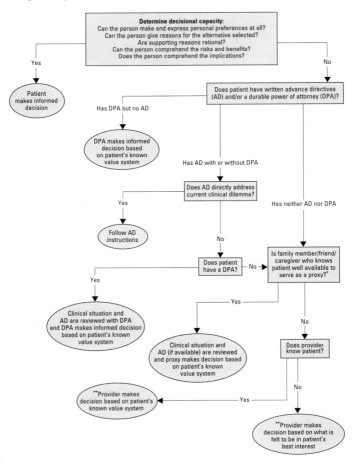

* State laws may dictate who is legal proxy.
** Or court-appointed decision maker (laws vary by state).

ELDER ABUSE
Risk Factors for Abuse of the Elderly Person
- Cognitive impairment
- Dependence of the abuser on the victim
- External factors causing stress
- History of violence
- Poor health and functional impairment
- Shared living arrangement
- Social isolation
- Substance abuse or mental illness on the part of the abuser

Source: Lachs MS, Pillemer K. Abuse and neglect of elderly persons. *N Engl J Med.* 1995;332(7):437–443.
Copyright © 1995 Massachusetts Medical Society. All rights reserved. Adapted with permission.

Presentations That Suggest Abuse or Neglect of an Elderly Patient
- Delays between an injury or illness and the seeking of medical attention
- Disparity in histories from the patient and the suspected abuser
- Implausible or vague explanations provided by either party
- Frequent visits to the emergency room for exacerbations of chronic disease despite a plan for medical care and adequate resources
- Presentation of a functionally impaired patient without his or her designated caregiver
- Laboratory findings that are inconsistent with the history provided

Source: Lachs MS, Pillemer K. Abuse and neglect of elderly persons. *N Engl J Med.* 1995;332(7):437–443. Copyright ©
1995 Massachusetts Medical Society. All rights reserved. Adapted with permission.

Questions To Ask About Possible Abuse
Many abuse victims can be identified simply by asking patients direct questions, eg:
- Has anyone at home ever hurt you?
- Are you afraid of anyone in your family?
- Has anyone ever scolded or threatened you?
- Are you receiving enough care at home?

Source: Jones JS. Abuse and neglect. In: Sanders AB, ed. *Emergency Care of the Elder Person.* St. Louis, MO: Beverly
Cracom Publications; 1996:181. Reprinted with permission.

If Abuse Is Suspected
- Perform further evaluation, including in-depth interview (often best accomplished by Adult Protective Services staff) and careful documentation of physical and psychologic findings.
- Report suspected abuse to Adult Protective Services; 42 states have mandatory reporting laws. (See p 230 for telephone numbers and Web sites.)

APPROPRIATE PRESCRIBING AND PHARMACOTHERAPY

HOW TO PRESCRIBE APPROPRIATELY AND AVOID POLYPHARMACY

- **Obtain a complete drug history.** Be sure to ask about previous treatments and responses as well as about other prescribers. Ask about allergies, OTC drugs, nutritional supplements, alternative medications, alcohol, tobacco, caffeine, and recreational drugs.
- **Avoid prescribing before a diagnosis is made.** Consider nondrug therapy. Eliminate drugs for which no diagnosis can be identified.
- **Review medications regularly and before prescribing a new medication.** Discontinue medications that have not had the intended response or are no longer needed. Monitor the use of prn and OTC drugs.
- **Know the actions, adverse effect and toxicity profiles of the medications you prescribe.** Consider how these might interact or complement existing drug therapy.
- **Start chronic drug therapy at a low dose and titrate dose on basis of tolerability and response.** Use drug levels when available.
- **Attempt to maximize dose before switching or adding another drug.** Encourage adherence with therapy. Educate patient and/or caregiver about each medication, its regimen, the therapeutic goal, its cost and potential adverse effects or drug interactions. Provide written instructions.
- **Avoid using one drug to treat the side effects of another.**
- **Attempt to use one drug to treat two or more conditions.**
- **Avoid combination products.**
- **Communicate with other prescribers.** Don't assume patients will—they assume you do!
- **Avoid using drugs from the same class or with similar actions** (eg, alprazolam and zolpidem).

For more on drugs that should be avoided in all elderly patients, see p 178.

WAYS TO IMPROVE PRESCRIPTION WRITING AND REDUCE MEDICATION ERRORS

- Be knowledgeable about the medication's dose, side effects, interactions, and monitoring.
- Write legibly to avoid misreading of the drug name (*Celexa* versus *Celebrex*).
- Write out the directions, strength, route, quantity, and number of refills.
- Always precede a decimal expression of <1 with a zero (0); never use a zero after a decimal.
- Avoid abbreviations, especially easily confused ones (qd and qid).
- Do not use ambiguous directions, eg, as directed (ud) or as needed.
- Include the medication's purpose in the directions (eg, for high blood pressure).
- Always re-read what you've written.

PHARMACOLOGIC THERAPY AND AGE-ASSOCIATED CHANGES

Parameter	Age Effect	Disease, Factor Effect	Prescribing Implications
Absorption	Rate and extent are usually unaffected	Achlorhydria, concurrent medications, tube feedings	Drug-drug and drug-food interactions are more likely to alter absorption
Distribution	Increase in fat : water ratio. Decreased plasma protein, particularly albumin	CHF, ascites, and other conditions will increase body water	Fat-soluble drugs have a larger volume of distribution. Highly protein-bound drugs will have a greater (active) free concentration
Metabolism	Decreases in liver mass and liver blood flow may decrease drug metabolism	Smoking, genotype, concurrent drug therapy, alcohol and caffeine intake may have more effect than aging	Lower doses may be therapeutic
Elimination	Primarily renal. Age-related decrease in GFR	Renal impairment with acute and chronic diseases; decreased muscle mass results in lower creatinine production	Serum creatinine not a reliable measure of renal function; best to estimate CrCl using formula on p 1
Pharmaco-dynamics	Less predictable and often altered drug response at usual or lower concentrations	Drug-drug and drug-disease interactions may alter responses	Prolonged pain relief with morphine at lower doses. Increased sedation and postural instability to benzodiazepines. Altered sensitivity to β-blockers

Table 5. Age-Associated Changes in Pharmacokinetics and Pharmacodynamics

AGGRAVATING FACTORS
Drug-Food or -Nutrient Interactions
Physical Interactions: Food or nutrients decrease or increase drug absorption (eg, products containing Mg^{++}, Ca^{++}, Fe^{++}, Al^{++}, or zinc can lower oral absorption of quinolone antibiotics, and tube feedings will decrease absorption of oral phenytoin and levothyroxine).

Decreased Drug Effect: Food or nutritional supplements can alter the intended pharmacologic response. The best example of this is warfarin and vitamin K-containing foods (eg, green leafy vegetables, broccoli, brussels sprout, greens, cabbage).

Decreased Oral Intake or Appetite: Drugs can alter the taste of food (dysgeusia) or decrease saliva production (xerostomia), making mastication and swallowing difficult. Drugs associated with dysgeusia include captopril and clarithromycin. Drugs that can cause xerostomia include antihistamines, antidepressants, antipsychotics, clonidine, and diuretics.

Drug-Drug Interactions
A drug's effect can be increased or decreased by another drug because of impaired absorption (eg, sucralfate and ciprofloxacin), displacement from protein-binding sites (eg, warfarin and sulfonamides), inhibition or induction of metabolic enzymes, or because two or more drugs have a similar pharmacologic effect (eg, potassium-sparing diuretics, potassium supplements, and ACE inhibitors). For drugs of particular concern, see **Table 6**.

Table 6. Selected CYP Isozyme Substrates, Inducers, and Inhibitors			
Substrates*	Isozyme	Inducers**	Inhibitors†
Acetaminophen Clozapine Desipramine Estradiol Imipramine Nortriptyline Olanzapine Warfarin	CYP1A2	Carbamazepine Cigarette smoke Omeprazole Phenobarbital Phenytoin Rifampin	Amiodarone Cimetidine Diltiazem Estradiol Fluoroquinolones Fluvoxamine Isoniazid Ketoconazole
Celecoxib Fluvastatin Phenytoin Warfarin	CYP2C9	Carbamazepine Phenobarbital Phenytoin Rifampin	Amiodarone Cimetidine Fluconazole Fluvoxamine Isoniazid Valproic acid
Codeine‡ Dextromethorphan Haloperidol Metoprolol Most TCAs Paroxetine Risperidone Timolol Tramadol‡ Venlafaxine	CYP2D6		Amiodarone Bupropion Celecoxib Cimetidine Diltiazem Fluoxetine Paroxetine Quinidine Valproic acid

Alprazolam
Amiodarone
Atorvastatin
Buspirone
Carbamazepine
Clarithromycin
Codeine
Cyclosporine
Dihydropyridine
  calcium channel
  blockers
Diltiazem
Erythromycin
Estradiol
Fluoxetine
Haloperidol
Itraconazole
Ketoconazole
Lovastatin
Nefazodone
Omeprazole
Pioglitazone
Quetiapine
Risperidone
Sildenafil
	CYP3A4	Carbamazepine
		Glucocorticoids
		Oxcarbazepine
		Phenobarbital
		Phenytoin
		Pioglitazone
		Rifabutin
		Rifampin
		St. John's wort
			Amiodarone
			Cimetidine
			Clarithromycin
			Cyclosporine
			Diltiazem
			Erythromycin
			Fluconazole
			Fluoxetine
			Fluvoxamine
			Grapefruit juice
			Haloperidol
			Isoniazid
			Itraconazole
			Ketoconazole
			Nefazodone
			Quinidine
			Sertraline
			Verapamil

Table 6. Selected CYP Isozyme Substrates, Inducers, and Inhibitors (cont.)			
Substrates*	**Isozyme**	**Inducers****	**Inhibitors†**
Simvastatin	CYP3A4 (cont.)		
Triazolam			
Venlafaxine			
Verapamil			
Warfarin			
Ziprasidone			
Zolpidem			

* Substrate: a drug metabolized by the isozyme.
** Inducer: a drug that increases the capacity of the isozyme to metabolize the substrate and potentially decreases the therapeutic effect.
† Inhibitor: a drug that prevents the isozyme from metabolizing the substrate and increases the risk for toxicity or therapeutic failure.
‡ Analgesic effect decreased because of inhibition of substrate metabolism to its active metabolite by an inhibitor.
Note: The list of medications is not comprehensive, but represents medications often prescribed for older patients or medications involved in very serious drug interactions (eg, cyclosporine). Some interactions have in vivo or in vitro documentation, whereas others are theoretical. For more information, consult a drug-drug interaction text or Internet resource, eg, http://medicine.iupui.edu/flockhart/.

Drug-Disease Interactions

Table 7. Drug-Disease Interactions		
Disease	**Drugs**	**Adverse Effects**
Benign prostatic hyperplasia	Anticholinergics, calcium channel blockers, decongestants	Urinary retention
Cardiac conduction abnormalities	Verapamil, TCAs, β-blockers (all routes)	Heart block
COPD or asthma	β-blockers (all routes), narcotic analgesics	Bronchoconstriction, respiratory depression
Chronic renal insufficiency	NSAIDs, contrast agents, aminoglycosides	Acute renal failure
Dementia	Anticholinergics, benzodiazepines, opiates, antidepressants, antiparkinsonian agents	Delirium
Diabetes mellitus	Diuretics, corticosteroids	Hyperglycemia
Angle-closure glaucoma	Anticholinergics	Acute ↑ in IOP
Hypertension	NSAIDs	Increased BP
Hypokalemia	Digoxin	Cardiac arrhythmias
Hyponatremia	Oral hypoglycemics, diuretics, SSRIs, carbamazepine, antipsychotics	↓ Serum sodium
Peptic ulcer	NSAIDs	Upper GI bleeding
Postural hypotension	Diuretics, TCAs, MAOIs, vasodilators, antiparkinsonian agents	Syncope, falls, hip fracture

Source: Adapted from Parker BM, Cusack BJ. Pharmacology and appropriate prescribing. In: Reuben DB, Yoshikawa TT, Besdine RW, eds. *Geriatrics Review Syllabus: A Core Curriculum in Geriatric Medicine.* 3rd ed. Dubuque, Iowa: Kendall/Hunt Publishing Company for the American Geriatrics Society; 1996:33. Reprinted with permission.

ALCOHOL ABUSE
Definition
Possible Alcohol Dependence—DSM-IV: Three or more of the following:
- Tolerance, requiring more alcohol to get "high"
- Withdrawal, or drinking to relieve, prevent withdrawal
- Drinking in larger amounts, or for a longer time than intended
- Persistent desire to drink, or unsuccessful efforts to control drinking
- Spending a lot of time obtaining, using alcohol, or recovering from effects
- Giving up important occupational, social, or recreational activities because of drinking
- Drinking despite persistent or recurrent physical or psychologic problems caused or worsened by alcohol

Possible Alcohol Abuse—DSM-IV: Recurring problems with one or more of the following:
- Drinking resulting in the failure to fulfill major obligations at work or in the home
- Drinking in situations where it is physically hazardous
- Alcohol-related legal problems
- Continued drinking despite social problems caused or worsened by alcohol

Hazardous Drinking: WHO definition—use of alcohol that places a person at risk of physical or psychologic complications. Increases risk of HTN (> 3 drinks/d), some cancers (eg, head and neck, esophagus, breast in women), and cirrhosis (higher in women). Possible increased risk for hip fracture and other injury. Multiple drug interactions, eg, antihypertensives, NSAIDs, H_2-blockers, sedatives, antidepressants.

Evaluation
Alcohol Misuse Screening: CAGE questionnaire has been validated in the older population.
C Have you ever felt you should **C**ut down?
A Does others' criticism of your drinking **A**nnoy you?
G Have you ever felt **G**uilty about drinking?
E Have you ever had an "**E**ye opener" to steady your nerves or get rid of a hangover?
  (*Positive response to any suggests problem drinking.*)

Detecting Harmful Drinking: May be missed by CAGE; ask
- How many days per week?
- How many drinks on those days?
- Maximum intake on any one day?
- What type (ie, beer, wine, or liquor)?
- What is in "a drink"?

  (≥ *2 drinks/d for women,* ≥ *3 drinks/d for men is potentially harmful.*)

Aggravating Factors
Alcohol Dependence or Abuse: Often missed in older persons because of reduced social and occupational functioning; signs more often are poor self-care, malnutrition, and medical illness.
Alcohol and Aging: Higher blood levels per amount consumed due to decreased lean body mass and total body water; concomitant medications may interact with alcohol.

Management

Alcohol Guidelines for Moderate Drinking: No more than 1 drink/d after age 65; 1 drink/d probably reduces cardiovascular risk.

Psychosocial Interventions:

- Problem drinking or alcohol misuse: Brief intervention; educate patient on effects of current drinking, point out current adverse effects.
- Alcohol dependence or abuse: Self-help groups (eg, Alcoholics Anonymous); professional (eg, psychodynamic, cognitive-behavioral, counseling, social support, family therapy, age-specific inpatient or outpatient).
- Drug therapy: See **Table 8.**
- Acute alcohol withdrawal: See p 36.

Table 8. Pharmacotherapy for Alcohol and Tobacco Abuse			
Drug	**Dosage**	**Formulations**	**Comment (Metabolism, Excretion)**
Alcohol Abuse			
Disulfiram (*Antabuse*)	125–500 mg qd	[T: 250, 500]	Not effective in clinical trials; serious cardiovascular side effects; multiple drug interactions (metabolism unknown)
✓ Naltrexone (*Depade*, *REVIA*, *Trexan*)	25 mg × 2d, then 50 mg qd max: 800 mg/d	[T: 50]	Monitor liver enzymes; useful adjunct to psychosocial therapy; contraindicated in renal failure; ~10% get nausea, headache (L, K)
Tobacco Abuse			
Bupropion (*Wellbutrin SR*, *Zyban*)	150 mg bid × 7–12 wk	[SR: 100, 150]	Combined with nicotine replacement, doubles quit rate to 30% at 12 mo; contraindicated with seizure disorders (L)
Nicotine Replacement*			
Transdermal patches** (eg, *Habitrol*, *Nicoderm*)	21 mg/d × 4–8 wk 14 mg/d × 2–4 wk 7 mg/d × 2–4 wk	[7, 14, 21]	Apply to clean, nonhairy skin on upper torso, rotate sites; start 14 mg/d with cardiovascular disease or body wt < 100 lb or if smoking < 10 cigarettes/d (L)
(*Nicotrol*)	15 mg/d × 6 wk 10 mg/d × 4–6 wk 5 mg/d × 4–6 wk	[5, 10, 15]	Gradually released over 16 h (L)
(*ProStep*)	22 mg/d × 4–8 wk 11 mg/d × 4–8 wk	[11, 22]	Persons < 100 lb start lower dose; reduce or D/C after 4–8 wk (L)
Polacrilex gum (*Nicorette*)	9–12 pieces/d	[2, 4]	Chew 1 piece when urge to smoke; usual 10–12 d, maximum 30/d; 4 mg for smokers > 21 cigarettes/d (L)
Nasal spray (*Nicotrol NS*)	1 spray each nostril q 30–60 min	[0.5 mg/spray]	Do not exceed 5 applications/h or 40 in 24 h (L)
Inhaler† (*Nicotrol Inhaler*)	6–16 cartridges/d	[4 mg delivered/cartridge]	Maximum 16 cartridges/d with gradual reduction after 6–12 wk if needed (L)

Note: ✓ = preferred for treating older persons.
* Best used in combination with smoking cessation program; dyspepsia is most common drug-related side effect.
** In patients receiving > 600 mg/d cimetidine, reduce to next lower patch dose.
† Available by prescription only.

ANTICOAGULATION

WARFARIN THERAPY

Prescribing Warfarin

- Usual dose of warfarin [*Coumadin, Carfin, Sofarin*] is 0.5–5.0 mg/d [T: 1, 2, 2.5, 3, 4, 5, 6, 7.5, 10] adjusted to achieve therapeutic INR (see **Table 9**).
- Initiate therapy by giving 2.0–5.0 mg/d as fixed dose; reduce dose if INR > 2.5 on day 3.
- Half-life is 31–51 h; steady state is achieved on day 5–7 of fixed dose.
- The following drugs **increase** INR in conjunction with warfarin: allopurinol, tamoxifen, omeprazole, propoxyphene, binge alcohol use, most antibiotics, NSAIDs, phenytoin, SSRIs, aspirin, amiodarone, corticosteroids, vitamin E (≥ 400 IU).
- The following drugs **decrease** INR in conjunction with warfarin: moderate alcohol use, cholestyramine, sucralfate, barbiturates, trazodone, carbamazepine, rifampin, estrogens, vitamin K.

Table 9. Anticoagulation Indicated in Absence of Active Bleeding or Severe Bleeding Risk		
Condition	Target INR	Duration of Therapy
Hip, major knee, and major gynecologic surgery	2.0–3.0	At least 3 mo or until patient is ambulatory
Symptomatic calf vein thrombosis	2.0–3.0	At least 3 mo
Proximal DVT	2.0–3.0	At least 6 mo
PE	2.0–3.0	6 mo
Recurrent thromboses or PE	2.0–3.0	Indefinitely
Atrial fibrillation	2.0–3.0	Indefinitely
Valvular heart disease with hx of systemic embolization or left atrial diameter > 5.5 cm	2.0–3.0	Indefinitely
Cardiomyopathy with EF < 25%	2.0–3.0	Indefinitely
Mechanical heart valve	2.5–3.5	Indefinitely
Prosthetic heart valve	2.5–3.5	3–6 mo
Acute MI complicated by severe LV dysfunction, CHF, previous emboli, mural thrombus on echocardiography	2.0–3.0	1–3 mo

Cessation of Anticoagulation Prior to Surgery

- If INR is between 2.0 and 3.0, hold warfarin 4 doses prior to surgery; longer if INR > 3.0.
- If patient has a mechanical valve, heparin should be used after warfarin is held prior to surgery.

Table 10. Treatment of Warfarin Overdose

INR	Clinical Situation	Action
> 3 and ≤ 6	No bleeding	Omit next few warfarin doses and restart at lower dose when INR ≤ 3.0
> 6 and ≤ 10.0	No bleeding	Omit next 2 doses of warfarin; give vitamin K (VK) 2.5 mg po
> 3 and ≤ 10.0	Minor bleeding or no bleeding but in need of rapid reversal for surgery	D/C warfarin; give VK 0.5–1.0 mg IV; repeat VK 0.5 mg IV after 24 h if INR > 3
> 3 and ≤ 10.0	Major bleeding	D/C warfarin; give VK 3–5 mg IV; check INR q 12 h; repeat VK 1–5 mg q 12 h if INR > 6; give fresh frozen plasma (FFP) as needed; consider hematology consult
> 10.0 and < 20.0	No bleeding	D/C warfarin; give VK 3–5 mg IV; check INR q 12 h; repeat VK 1–5 mg q 12 h if INR > 6
> 10.0 and < 20.0	Bleeding	Same as above + FFP; obtain hematology consult
≥ 20.0	No bleeding	D/C warfarin; give VK 10 mg IV; check INR q 6 h; repeat VK q 12 h as needed; observe very closely for bleeding
≥ 20.0	Bleeding	D/C warfarin, give VK 10–25 mg IV + FFP; obtain hematology consult

Source: Adapted from Lacy CF, Armstrong LL, Goldman MP, Lance LL. *Drug Information Handbook*, 7th ed. Hudson (Cleveland, OH): Lexi-Comp, Inc.; 1999:1229. Reprinted with permission.

ACUTE ANTICOAGULATION

Table 11. Weight-Based Heparin Dosage

Initial	80 U/kg bolus = _____ U (not to exceed 10,000 U) 18 U/kg/h = _____ U/h (not to exceed 1500 U)
PTT < 35	80 U/kg bolus = _____ U Increase drip 4 U/kg/h = _____ U/h
PTT 35 to 45	40 U/kg bolus = _____ U Increase drip 2 U/kg/h = _____ U/h
PTT 46 to 70	No change
PTT 71 to 90	Reduce drip to 2 U/kg/h = _____ U/h Hold heparin for 1 h Reduce drip 3 U/kg/h = _____ U/h

Note: Order PTT 6 h after any dosage change, adjusting heparin infusion by the sliding scale until PTT is therapeutic (46–70 sec). When two consecutive PTTs are therapeutic, order PTT (and readjust heparin drip as needed) q 24 h.
Source: Adapted from Figure 3 in Raschke RA, Reilly BM, Guidry JR, et al. Weight-based heparin dosing nomogram compared with a standard care nomogram. *Ann Intern Med*. 1993;119(9):874. Reprinted with permission.

Table 12. Other Anticoagulants

Agent	Dosage	Half-Life	Comments (Metabolism, Excretion)
Low-molecular-weight heparins: doses are for treatment, NOT prevention of DVT			
Enoxaparin (*Lovenox*)	1 mg/kg SC q 12 h *or* 1.5 mg/kg qd	3–6 h	Bleeding, anemia, hyperkalemia, hypertransaminasemia, thrombocytopenia, thrombocytosis, urticaria, angioedema (K)
Dalteparin (*Fragmin*)	100 anti-Xa units/ kg SC q 12 h *or* 200 anti-X units/kg qd	3–4 h	Same (K)
Tinzaparin (*Innohep*)	175 anti-Xa IU/kg SC qd	3–4 h	Same (K)
Thrombolytic therapy: doses are for treatment of massive PE			
Streptokinase (*Kabikinase, Streptase*)	250,000 μ over 30 min and 100,000 μ/h × 24 h	1.3 h	Risk of hemorrhage ↑ with age and higher BMI; hypotension, hallucination, agitation, confusion, serum sickness (L)
Urokinase (*Abbokinase*)	4400 IU/kg in 15 mL D5W or NS over 20 min and q 12 h, not to exceed 200 mL	20 min	Hemorrhage, fever, platelet aggregation (L)

ANXIETY

DIAGNOSIS
Anxiety disorders are less prevalent in elderly than in younger adults. New-onset anxiety in elderly persons is often secondary to physical illness, depression, medication side effects, or withdrawal from drugs.

DSM-IV recognizes several anxiety disorders:
(***Bold** type indicates the most common anxiety disorders occurring in older persons.*)
• Acute stress disorder
• Agoraphobia without a history of panic
• **GAD, anxiety disorder due to a general medical condition**
• Obsessive-compulsive disorder (OCD)
• Panic disorder, with or without agoraphobia
• Posttraumatic stress disorder
• Social phobia
• Specific phobia
• Substance-induced anxiety disorder

DSM-IV Criteria for GAD
• Excessive anxiety and worry on more days than not for ≥ 6 mo, about a number of events or activities
• Difficulty controlling the worry
• Anxiety and worry associated with ≥ 3 of 6 symptoms:
   - restlessness or feeling keyed up or on edge
   - being easily fatigued
   - difficulty concentrating or mind going blank
   - irritability
   - muscle tension
   - sleep disturbance (difficulty falling or staying asleep, or restless unsatisfying sleep)
• Focus of anxiety and worry not confined to features of an Axis I disorder (primary psychiatric disorder); often, about routine life circumstances; may shift from one concern to another
• Anxiety, worry, or physical symptoms cause clinically significant distress or impairment in social, occupational, or other important areas of functioning
• Disturbance not due to the direct physiologic effects of a drug of abuse or a medication or to a medical condition; does not occur exclusively during a mood disorder, psychotic disorder, or a pervasive development disorder.

DSM-IV Criteria for Panic Attack

Discrete period of intense fear or discomfort with ≥ 4 of the following (also, must peak within 10 min):

- Palpitations, rapid HR
- Sweating
- Trembling or shaking
- Sensations of SOB or smothering
- Choking feeling
- Chest pain or discomfort
- Nausea or abdominal distress
- Feeling dizzy, unsteady, lightheaded, or faint
- Feelings of unreality or being detached from self
- Fear of losing control or going crazy
- Fear of dying
- Paresthesias
- Chills or hot flushes

Differential Diagnosis

- Physical conditions producing anxiety
  - Cardiovascular: Arrhythmias, angina, MI, CHF
  - Endocrine: Hyperthyroidism, hypoglycemia, pheochromocytoma
  - Neurologic: Movement disorders, temporal lobe epilepsy, AD, stroke
  - Respiratory: COPD, asthma, pulmonary embolism
- Medications producing anxiety
  - Caffeine
  - Corticosteroids
  - Nicotine
  - Psychotropics: Antidepressants, antipsychotics, stimulants
  - Sympathomimetics: Pseudoephedrine, β-agonists
  - Thyroid hormones: Overreplacement
- Withdrawal states: alcohol, sedatives, hypnotics, benzodiazepines
- Depression

EVALUATION

- Past psychiatric history
- Drug review: Prescribed, OTC, alcohol, caffeine
- Mental status evaluation
- Physical examination: Focus on signs and symptoms of anxiety (eg, tachycardia, hyperpnea, sweating, tremor)
- Laboratory tests: Consider CBC, blood glucose, TSH, B_{12}, ECG, oxygen saturation, drug and alcohol screening

MANAGEMENT

Nonpharmacologic

Cognitive-behavior therapy (CBT) may be useful for GAD, panic disorder, and OCD. May be effective alone but mostly used in conjunction with pharmacotherapy. CBT requires a cognitively intact, motivated patient.

Pharmacologic

- Recommended initial treatments for GAD are paroxetene or venlafaxine.
- SSRIs are initial treatment for OCD and panic disorder. (See **Table 23.**)
- Secondary treatments for OCD and panic disorder may include β-blockers and atypical antipsychotics.

Antidepressants Approved for Anxiety Disorders: See **Table 23** for dosing.
- Obsessive-compulsive: fluoxetine, fluvoxamine, paroxetine, sertraline
- Panic: sertraline, paroxetine
- Social phobia: paroxetine
- Generalized anxiety: venlafaxine, paroxetine
- Post-traumatic stress: sertraline

***Buspirone* (BuSpar):**
- Serotonin 1A partial agonist effective in GAD and anxiety symptoms accompanying general medical illness
- Not effective for acute anxiety, panic, or OCD
- May take 2–4 wk for therapeutic response
- Recommended geriatric dosage: 15–20 mg bid [T: 5, 10, 15, 30]
- No dependence, tolerance, withdrawal, CNS depression, or significant drug-drug interactions

Benzodiazepines:
- Most often used for acute anxiety, GAD, panic, OCD
- Preferred: Intermediate–half-life drugs inactivated by direct conjugation in liver and therefore less affected by aging

Table 13. Benzodiazepines for Anxiety Recommended for Geriatric Patients		
Drug	**Dosage**	**Formulations**
Lorazepam (*Ativan*)	0.5–2 mg in 2–3 divided doses	[T: 0.5, 1, 2; S: 2 mg/mL; Inj: 2mg/mL]
Oxazepam (*Serax*)	10–15 mg bid–tid	[T: 10, 15, 30]

- Long-acting benzodiazepines (eg, flurazepam, diazepam, chlordiazepoxide): Linked to cognitive impairment, falls, sedation, psychomotor impairment
- Problems: Dependence, tolerance, withdrawal, more so with short-acting benzodiazepines; seizure risk with alprazolam withdrawal
- Potentially fatal if combined with alcohol or other CNS depressants
- Only short-term (60–90 d) use recommended

CARDIOVASCULAR DISEASES

DIAGNOSTIC CARDIAC TESTS
Angina, Coronary Artery Disease
- Cardiac catheterization is the gold standard.
- Stress testing: The heart is stressed either through exercise (treadmill, stationary bicycle) or, if the patient cannot exercise or the ECG is markedly abnormal, with pharmacologic agents (dipyridamole, adenosine, dobutamine). Exercise stress tests can be performed with or without cardiac imaging, while pharmacologic stress tests always include imaging. Imaging can be accomplished by a nuclear isotope (eg, thallium) or echocardiography.
- Cardiac enzymes if acute chest pain (troponin, CPK)
- Electron-beam computed tomography (EBCT) is not currently recommended as a screening test for CAD.

Congestive Heart Failure
- First line: ECG, CXR, echocardiogram (provides valuable information about left ventricular size and function, valvular function; difficult to perform in patients with obesity or lung disease)
- Other: Radionuclide ventriculography (which measures EF more precisely, provides a better evaluation of right ventricular function, and is more expensive than echocardiography)

Palpitations, Presyncope, Syncope
- First line: CXR, ECG, 24- or 48-h rhythm (Holter) monitoring
- Other: Ambulatory BP monitoring, tilt-table testing

ACUTE MYOCARDIAL INFARCTION
Evaluation and Assessment
- As in younger persons, diagnosis is made by cardiac enzyme rises, with or without ECG changes.
- Both creatine kinase MB isoenzymes (CK-MB) and cardiac troponins T and I usually become elevated 4 h following myocardial injury.
- Elevated troponin in the face of normal CK-MB can indicate increased risk of MI in the ensuing 6 mo.
- Troponins are not useful for detecting reinfarction within 1st wk of an MI. CK-MB is the preferred marker for early reinfarction.
- CK-MB subforms are the most sensitive and specific test for detecting MI in the first 6 h, but troponin remains elevated longer.
- Both CK-MB and cardiac troponins can exhibit false-positive results that are due to subclinical ischemic myocardial injury or nonischemic myocardial injury.
- Serial enzyme measurements are necessary to exclude MI.
- Presentation frequently atypical—suspect MI with atypical chest pain; arm, jaw, or abdominal pain (with or without nausea); acute functional decline.

- Risk factors for acute MI in older adults:

Strong:
- Previous MI or angina
- Age
- Diabetes mellitus
- Hypertension
- Smoking
- Severe coronary artery calcification

Weak:
- Dyslipidemia (except in those with overt coronary disease)
- Family history
- Obesity
- Sedentary life style

Management

Thrombolytic Therapy for Q-wave MI (Chest Pain < 12 h, ≥ 1 mm ST-Segment Elevation):
- Age is not a contraindication.
- Absolute contraindications (ACC/AHA):
- Prior hemorrhagic stroke
- Other stroke or intracerebral event in past yr
- Active internal bleeding
- Known intracranial neoplasm
- Aortic dissection
- Relative contraindications:
- BP > 180/110 on presentation
- History of prior stroke or known intracerebral pathology not covered in absolute contraindications
- Current therapeutic INR ≥ 3
- Known bleeding diathesis
- Recent (< 3 wk) major surgery
- Prolonged (> 10 min) or traumatic CPR
- Recent (< 2–4 wk) trauma or internal bleeding
- Noncompressible vascular puncture
- Active peptic ulcer
- History of severe, chronic HTN
- For streptokinase or anistreplase, prior exposure (5 d–2 yr) or prior allergic reactions

Surgery: Percutaneous transluminal coronary angioplasty (PTCA) or emergent coronary artery bypass grafting (CABG) are alternatives to thrombolytic therapy.

Pharmacologic Management: For both Q-wave MI and acute coronary syndrome (unstable angina or non-Q-wave MI)
- Aspirin, at least 160 mg qd initially, should be started at the time of MI and continued indefinitely at 81–325 mg/d.
- In addition to aspirin therapy, clopidogrel (*Plavix*) 300 mg po initially followed by 75 mg po qd [T:75] can lower risk of recurrent MI; combination therapy with acetylsalicylic acid (ASA) and clopidogrel is also associated with higher bleeding complications, so therapy should be considered only for those at low bleeding risk.
- Heparin should be given acutely. For patients undergoing thrombolytic therapy or immediate PTCA, those with continuing pain or those with indications for warfarin therapy (see below), give 5000 units bolus IV + 1000 units/h IV; check activated PTT q 6 h (target 1.5–2.0 × control). Otherwise, give 7500 units SC q 12 h until patient is fully ambulatory.
- β-Blockers should be given acutely and continued chronically unless systolic failure or pronounced bradycardia is present. Acute phase: Atenolol (*Tenormin*), 5 mg IV over 5 min and repeat in 10 min; or metoprolol (*Lopressor*) 5 mg IV q 5 min up to a total of 15 mg. Begin chronic phase within 1–2 h: atenolol 25–100 mg po qd or metoprolol, 50–200 mg po bid.
- Oxygen: 2–4 L/min via nasal cannula should be given acutely.
- Nitroglycerin is indicated acutely for persistent ischemia, hypertension, or CHF. Begin at 5–10 μg/min IV and titrate to pain relief, SBP > 90, or resolution of ECG abnormalities.

- ACE inhibitors should be started within 1st 24 h following MI with ST-segment elevation, particularly in cases with systolic dysfunction, eg: captopril (*Capoten*), 6.25–25 mg po bid–tid; enalapril (*Vasotec*), 2.5–20 mg po qd/bid; lisinopril (*Prinivil, Zestril*), 2.5–20 mg po qd.
- Warfarin therapy is indicated in post-MI patients with atrial fibrillation, left ventricular thrombosis, or large anterior infarction (see **Table 9**).
- Lipid-lowering therapy (see Dyslipidemia, p 24) to achieve target levels (total cholesterol < 160 mg/dL, LDL cholesterol < 100 mg/dL, HDL cholesterol > 45 mg/dL) should be initiated by the time of hospital discharge.
- At time of discharge, prescribe rapid-acting nitrates prn. Sublingual nitroglycerin or nitroglycerin spray every 5 min for maximum of 3 doses in 15 min. See **Table 14**.
- Calcium channel blockers should be used cautiously, only in non-Q-wave infarctions without systolic dysfunction and a contraindication to β-blockers.
- Longer-acting nitrates if symptomatic angina and treatment will be medical rather than surgical or angioplasty. May be combined with β-blockers or calcium channel blockers, or both. See **Table 14**.
- Patients with hematocrit ≤ 30 and who are hemodynamically stable should be transfused to achieve hematocrit > 33.

Table 14. Nitrate Dosages and Formulations		
Drug	**Dosage**	**Formulations**
Oral		
Isosorbide dinitrate (*Isordil, Sorbitrate*)	10–40 mg tid (6 h apart)	[T: 5, 10, 20, 30, 40; CT: 5, 10]
Isosorbide dinitrate SR (*Isordil Tembids, Dilatrate SR*)	40–80 mg bid–tid	[T: 40]
Isosorbide mononitrate (*ISMO, Monoket*)	20 mg bid (8 AM and 3 PM)	[T: 10, 20]
Isosorbide mononitrate SR (*Imdur*)	start 30–60 mg qd; max 240 mg/d	[T: 30, 60, 120]
Nitroglycerin (*Nitro-Bid*)	2.5–9 mg bid–tid	[T: 2.5, 6.5, 9]
Sublingual		
Isosorbide dinitrate (*Isordil, Sorbitrate*)	1 tablet prn	[T: 2.5, 5, 10]
Nitroglycerin (*Nitrostat*)	0.4 mg prn	[T: 0.15, 0.3, 0.4, 0.6]
Oral spray		
Nitroglycerin (*Nitrolingual*)	1–2 sprays prn; max 3/15 min	[0.4 mg/spray]
Ointment		
Nitroglycerin 2% (*Nitro-Bid, Nitrol*)	start 0.5–4 inches q 4–8 h	[2%]
Transdermal		
Nitroglycerin (*Deponit*) (*Minitran*) (*Nitrek*) (*Nitro-Dur*) (*Nitrodisc*) (*Transderm-Nitro*)	1 patch 12–14 h/d	[0.2, 0.4 (mg/h)] [0.1, 0.2, 0.4, 0.6] [0.2, 0.4, 0.6 (mg/h)] [0.1, 0.2, 0.3, 0.4, 0.6, 0.8] [0.2, 0.3, 0.4] [0.1, 0.2, 0.4, 0.6, 0.8]

CONGESTIVE HEART FAILURE
Evaluation and Assessment
- All patients initially presenting with CHF should have an echocardiogram to evaluate left ventricular function. An ejection fraction (EF) of < 40% indicates systolic dysfunction. Heart failure with an EF ≥ 40% indicates diastolic dysfunction.
- Other routine assessment tests: ECG, CXR, CBC, electrolytes, creatinine, albumin, LFTs, TSH, UA
- New York Heart Association (NYHA) classification of cardiac disability:
- Class I—cardiac disease without resulting limitation of physical activity
- Class II—comfortable at rest, but symptoms (dyspnea, fatigue, palpitation, angina) on normal physical activity
- Class III—comfortable at rest, but symptoms on slight physical activity
- Class IV—symptoms at rest

Management*
Nonpharmacologic:
- Exercise: Regular walking or cycling for NYHA Class I–III disability
- Measure weight daily
- Salt restriction: 3 g sodium diet is reasonable goal; 2 g in severe CHF

Pharmacologic: For information on drug dosages and side effects not listed below, see **Table 16**.
- Systolic dysfunction:
- Diuretics if volume overload
- ACE inhibitors to target levels, eg, 150 mg/d of captopril or ≥ 20 mg/d of enalapril or lisinopril
- Add digoxin (*Lanoxin*) [T: 0.125, 0.25; S: 0.05 mg/mL]; (*Lanoxicaps*) [T: 0.05, 0.1, 0.2], 0.125–0.375 mg qd (monitor serum levels) if CHF is not controlled on diuretics and ACE inhibitors. The following **increase** digoxin concentration or effect, or both: quinidine, indomethacin, verapamil, nifedipine, diltiazem, esmolol, flecainide, hydroxychloroquine, ibuprofen, quinine, tolbutamide, amiodarone, erythromycin, tetracycline, and spironolactone. The following **decrease** digoxin concentration or effect, or both: antacids, psyllium, kaolin-pectin, aminosalicylic acid, colestipol, sulfasalazine, antineoplastics, cholestyramine, metoclopramide, and St. John's wort.
- For patients with NYHA Class II or III failure, a β-blocker (metoprolol XL [*Toprol-XL*] 12.5–25 mg po qd initially, maximum 200 mg/d; or bisoprolol [*Zebeta*] 1.25 mg po qd initially, maximum 5 mg qd) or carvedilol (*Coreg*) 3.125 mg po bid initially, maximum 25 mg bid should be added for long-term CHF management if there is no contraindication to β-blockers (do not add β-blockers in acutely ill patients).
- For patients with NYHA Class III or IV failure and creatinine < 2.5 mg/dL, addition of spironolactone (*Aldactone*) 25 mg qd [T: 25] can reduce mortality; follow serum potassium.
- Many clinicians recommend anticoagulating patients with EF < 25% (see **Table 9**).
- Calcium channel blockers, class I antiarrhythmics, hydralazine, and nitroglycerin are not indicated.
- Diastolic dysfunction:
- Diuretics should be used judiciously and only if there is volume overload.
- There is no agreed-upon primary treatment of diastolic dysfunction. β-Blockers, ACE inhibitors, and/or non-dihydropyridine calcium channel blockers may be of benefit.

* Source: Consensus recommendations for the management of chronic heart failure. *Am J Cardiol.* 1999;83(2A):1A–38A.

DYSLIPIDEMIA
Treatment Indications
- Older adults should have dyslipidemia treated if they have overt atherosclerotic disease: CHD (angina, previous MI), peripheral arterial disease, abdominal aortic aneurysm, or symptomatic carotid artery disease (TIA or prior stroke). Treatment goal is LDL < 100 mg/dL.
- National Cholesterol Education Program recommends treating diabetes as CHD risk equivalent. Treatment goal is LDL < 100 mg/dL.
- Dyslipidemia treatment should be considered in older adults without overt atherosclerotic disease or diabetes, but with multiple other CHD risk factors (HTN, smoking, family history of premature CHD, HDL < 40 mg/dL, male sex). In general, treatment goals are LDL < 130 mg/dL for 2+ risk factors and < 160 mg/dL for 0–1 risk factors. However, more severe individual risk factor profiles may indicate the need for a lower LDL level treatment goal. See www.nhlbi.nih.gov.

Management
Nonpharmacologic: A cholesterol-lowering diet should be considered initial therapy for dyslipidemia and should be used as follows:
- The patient should be at low risk for malnutrition.
- The diet should be nutritionally adequate, with sufficient total calories, protein, calcium, iron, and vitamins.
- The diet should be easily understood and affordable (a dietitian can be very helpful).
- Cholesterol-lowering margarines can lower LDL cholesterol by 10% to 15% (*Take Control* 1–2 tablespoons/d; *Benecol* 3 servings [1.5 teaspoons]/d).

Pharmacologic: Target drug treatment according to type of dyslipidemia.

Table 15. Drug Regimens for Dyslipidemia			
Condition	**Drug**	**Dosage**	**Formulations**
Elevated LDL, normal TG	HMG-CoA reductase inhibitor*		
	Atorvastatin (*Lipitor*)	10–80 mg qd	[T: 10, 20, 40]
	Fluvastatin (*Lescol*)	20–80 mg qd in P.M., max 80 mg	[C: 20, 40; T: ER 80]
	Lovastatin (*Mevacor*)	10–40 mg qd–bid	[T: 10, 20, 40]
	Pravastatin (*Pravachol*)	10–40 mg qd	[T: 10, 20]
	Simvastatin (*Zocor*)	5–80 mg qd in P.M.	[T: 5, 10, 20, 40, 80]
Elevated TG (> 500 mg/dL)	Gemfibrozil (*Lopid*)	300–600 mg po bid	[T: 600]

Table 15. Drug Regimens for Dyslipidemia (cont.)			
Condition	**Drug**	**Dosage**	**Formulations**
Combined elevated LDL, low HDL, elevated TG	Gemfibrozil, HMG-CoA (if TG < 300 mg/dL), conjugated estrogen (in women, see p 160)	as above	as above
Alternative for any of above	Niacin[†]	100 mg tid to start; increase to 500–1000 mg tid	[T: 25, 50, 100, 250, 500, ER or TR 150, 250, 500, 750, 1000; C: TR 125, 250, 400, 500]

* Monitor CPK and transaminases q 3 mo for 1 yr, watch for myopathy at higher doses or when used with another antidyslipidemic drug. Should be taken in the evening.

[†] Monitor for flushing, pruritus, nausea, gastritis, ulcer. Aspirin 325 mg po 30 min prior to first niacin dose of the day is quite effective in preventing side effects.

HYPERTENSION
Definition, Classification
JNC-VI defines HTN as SBP > 140 or DBP > 90. In elderly persons, many clinicians define HTN as SBP > 160 or DBP > 90. Isolated systolic HTN (SBP > 160 with DBP < 90) should be vigorously treated.

Evaluation and Assessment
• Measure both standing and sitting BP after 5 min of rest.
• Base diagnosis on two or more readings at each of two or more visits. Once diagnosis is made, evaluation includes:
- Assessment of cardiac risk factors: smoking, dyslipidemia, and diabetes mellitus are important in older adults.
- Assessment of end-organ damage: LVH, angina, prior MI, prior coronary revascularization, CHF, stroke or TIA, nephropathy, peripheral arterial disease, retinopathy.
- Routine laboratory tests: CBC, UA, electrolytes, creatinine, fasting glucose, total cholesterol, HDL cholesterol, and ECG.
- Think renal artery stenosis if sudden onset of HTN, sudden rise in BP in previously well-controlled HTN, or HTN despite treatment with three antihypertensives.

Aggravating Factors
Almost all are related to life style:
• Emotional stress
• Excessive alcohol intake
• Excessive salt intake
• Lack of aerobic exercise
• Low potassium intake
• Low calcium intake
• Nicotine
• Obesity

Management
(JNC-VI recommendations). Lowering BP below 120/80 is not recommended.
Nonpharmacologic:
• Adequate calcium and magnesium intake as well as a low-fat diet are recommended for optimizing general health.
• Adequate dietary potassium intake; fruits and vegetables are the best sources.
• Aerobic exercise—30–45 min most days of the week—is recommended.
• Moderation of alcohol intake—limit to 1 oz of ethanol/d.

- Moderation of dietary sodium: watch for volume depletion with diuretic use.
- Smoking cessation
- Weight reduction: even a 10-lb weight loss can significantly lower BP.

Pharmacologic:
Table 16 lists commonly used antihypertensives.
- Use antihypertensives carefully in patients with orthostatic BP drop; base treatment decisions on standing BP.
- In the absence of coexisting conditions, a thiazide diuretic or β-blocker can be used as a first-line drug.
- In the presence of coexisting conditions, therapy should be individualized (see **Table 17**).
- Antihypertensive combinations are listed in **Table 18.**
- Available dose formulations of oral potassium supplements: [T: (mEq) 6, 7, 8, 10, 20; S: (mEq/15 mL) 20, 40; powders (mEq/pack) l5, 20, 25]

Hypertensive Emergencies and Urgencies:
- Elevated BP alone without symptoms or target end organ damage rarely requires emergent BP lowering.
- Conditions requiring emergent BP lowering include hypertensive encephalopathy, intracranial hemorrhage, unstable angina, acute MI, acute LV failure with pulmonary edema, dissecting aortic aneurysm.
- Most common initial treatment for emergent BP lowering is sodium nitroprusside (*Nipride*) 0.25–10 mg/kg/min as IV infusion.
- For nonemergent (ie, urgent) BP lowering, give a standard dose of a recommended antihypertensive orally (see **Table 16**) or an extra dose of the patient's usual oral antihypertensive.

Table 16. Oral Antihypertensive Agents			
Class, Drug	**Geriatric Dose Range, total mg/d (times/d)**	**Formulations**	**Comments (Metabolism, Excretion)**
Diuretics			↓ potassium, Na, magnesium levels; ↑ uric acid, calcium, cholesterol (mild) and glucose (mild) levels
Thiazides			
✓ Chlorthalidone (*Hygroton*)	12.5–25 (1)	[T: 15, 25, 50, 100]	Increased side effects at > 25 mg/d (L)
✓ Hydrochlorothiazide (*Esidrix, HydroDIURIL, Oretic*)	12.5–25 (1)	[T: 25, 50, 100; S: 50 mg/mL; C: 12.5]	Increased side effects at > 25 mg/d (L)
✓ Indapamide (*Lozol*)	0.625–2.5 (1)	[T: 1.25, 2.5]	Less or no hypercholesterolemia (L)
Metolazone (*Mykrox*)	0.25–0.5 (1)	[T rapid: 0.5]	Monitor electrolytes carefully (L)

Note: Listing of side effects is not exhaustive, and side effects are for the class of drugs except where noted for individual drugs. ✓ = preferred antihypertensive agent for treating older persons; ♥ = useful in treating heart failure.

Class, Drug	Geriatric Dose Range, total mg/d (times/d)	Formulations	Comments (Metabolism, Excretion)
Metolazone (Zaroxolyn)	2.5–5 (1)	[T: 2.5, 5, 10]	Monitor electrolytes carefully (L)
Loop diuretics ♥ Bumetanide (Bumex)	0.5–4 (1–3)	[T: 0.5, 1, 2]	Short duration of action, no hypercalcemia (K)
♥ Ethacrynic acid (Edecrin)	12.5–50 (1–3)	[T: 25, 50]	Only nonsulfonamide diuretic, ototoxicity (K)
♥ Furosemide (Lasix)	20–160 (1–2)	[T: 20, 40, 80; S: 10, 40 mg/5 mL]	Short duration of action, no hypercalcemia (K)
♥ Torsemide (Demadex)	2.5–50 (1–2)	[T: 5, 10, 20, 100; Inj.]	Short duration of action, no hypercalcemia (K)
Potassium-sparing drugs Amiloride (Midamor)	2.5–10 (1)	[T: 5]	(L, K)
♥ Spironolactone (Aldactone)	12.5–50 (1–2)	[T: 25, 50, 100]	Gynecomastia; appropriate at 25 mg dose in NYHA Class III or IV CHF (L, K)
Triamterene (Dyrenium)	25–100 (1–2)	[T: 50, 100]	(L, K)
Adrenergic Inhibitors α-Blockers			Avoid as primary therapy for HTN unless patient has BPH
Doxazosin (Cardura)	1–16 (1)	[T: 1, 2, 4, 8]	(L)
Prazosin (Minipress)	1–30 (2–3)	[T: 1, 2, 5]	(L)
Terazosin (Hytrin)	1–20 (1)	[T: 1, 2, 5, 10; C: 1, 2, 5, 10]	(L, K)
Peripheral agents Guanadrel (Hylorel)	5–50 (2)	[T: 10, 25]	Postural hypotension, diarrhea (K)
Guanethidine (Ismelin)	5–25 (1)	[T: 10, 25]	Postural hypotension, diarrhea (L, K)
Reserpine (Serpasil)	0.05–0.25 (1)	[T: 0.1, 0.25]	Sedation, depression, nasal congestion, activation of peptic ulcer (L, K)

Table 16. Oral Antihypertensive Agents (cont.)

Note: Listing of side effects is not exhaustive, and side effects are for the class of drugs except where noted for individual drugs. ✓ = preferred antihypertensive agent for treating older persons; ♥ = useful in treating heart failure.

(continues)

Table 16. Oral Antihypertensive Agents (cont.)

Class, Drug	Geriatric Dose Range, total mg/d (times/d)	Formulations	Comments (Metabolism, Excretion)
Central α-agonists			Sedation, dry mouth, bradycardia, withdrawal hypertension
Clonidine (*Catapres, Catapres-TTS*)	0.1–1.2 (2–3 or patch 1/wk)	[T: 0.1, 0.2, 0.3; patch: 0.1, 0.2, 0.3 mg/d]	(L, K)
Guanabenz (*Wytensin*)	4–16 (2)	[T: 4, 8]	(L, K)
Guanfacine (*Tenex*)	0.5–2 (1)	[T: 1, 2]	(K)
Methyldopa (*Aldomet*)	250–2500 (2)	[T: 125, 250, 500; S: 250 mg/5 mL]	(L, K)
β-Blockers			Bronchospasm, bradycardia, acute heart failure, may mask insulin-induced hypoglycemia
✓ Acebutolol (*Sectral*)	200–800 (1)	[C: 200, 400]	$β_1$, low lipid solubility (L, K)
✓ Atenolol (*Tenormin*)	12.5–100 (1)	[T: 25, 50, 100]	$β_1$, low lipid solubility (K)
✓ Betaxolol (*Kerlone*)	5–20 (1)	[T: 10, 20]	$β_1$, low lipid solubility (L, K)
✓ ♥ Bisoprolol (*Zebeta*)	2.5–10 (1)	[T: 5, 10]	$β_1$, low lipid solubility (L, K)
✓ Carteolol (*Cartrol*)	1.25–10 (1)	[T: 2.5, 5]	$β_1$, low lipid solubility (K)
✓ Metoprolol (*Lopressor*)	25–400 (2)	[T: 50, 100]	$β_1$, moderate lipid solubility (L)
✓ ♥ Long-acting (*Toprol XL*)	50–400 (1)	[T: 25, 50, 100, 200]	(L)
Nadolol (*Corgard*)	20–160 (1)	[T: 20, 40, 80, 120, 160]	$β_1$, $β_2$, low lipid solubility (K)
Penbutolol (*Levatol*)	10–20 (1)	[T: 20]	$β_1$, $β_2$, high lipid solubility (L, K)
Pindolol (*Visken*)	5–60 (2)	[T: 5, 10]	$β_1$, $β_2$, moderate lipid solubility (K)
Propranolol (*Inderal*)	20–360 (2)	[T: 10, 20, 40, 60, 80, 90; S: 4/mL, 8/mL]	$β_1$, $β_2$, high lipid solubility (L)
Long-acting (*Inderal LA*)	60–320 (1)	[C: 60, 80, 120, 160]	(L)
Timolol (*Blocadren*)	10–60 (2)	[T: 5, 10, 20]	$β_1$, $β_2$, low to moderate lipid solubility (L, K)
Combined α- and β-Blockers			Postural hypotension, bronchospasm
✓ ♥ Carvedilol (*Coreg*)	3.125–25 (2)	[T: 3.125, 6.25, 12.5, 25]	$β_1$, $β_2$, high lipid solubility (L)

Note: Listing of side effects is not exhaustive, and side effects are for the class of drugs except where noted for individual drugs. ✓ = preferred antihypertensive agent for treating older persons; ♥ = useful in treating heart failure.

Table 16. Oral Antihypertensive Agents (cont.)

Class, Drug	Geriatric Dose Range, total mg/d (times/d)	Formulations	Comments (Metabolism, Excretion)
✓ Labetalol (*Normodyne, Trandate*)	100–600 (2)	[T: 100, 200, 300]	β_1, β_2, moderate lipid solubility (L, K)
Direct Vasodilators			Headaches, fluid retention, tachycardia
Hydralazine (*Apresoline*)	40–200 (2–4)	[T: 10, 25, 50, 100; Inj.]	Lupus syndrome (L, K)
Minoxidil (*Loniten*)	2.5–50 (1)	[T: 2.5, 10]	Hirsutism (K)
Calcium Antagonists			
Nondihydropyridines			Conduction defects, worsening of systolic dysfunction, gingival hyperplasia
✓ Diltiazem SR (*Cardizem CD, Cardizem SR, Dilacor XR, Tiazac*)	120–360 (1–2) max 480	[C: 1/d: 120, 180, 240, 300, 360, 420; 2/d: 60, 90, 120; T: 30, 60, 90, 120; ER 120, 180, 240]	Nausea, headache (L)
✓ Verapamil SR (*Calan SR, Covera-HS, Isoptin SR, Verelan*)	120–480 (1–2)	[T: SR 120, 180, 240; C: SR 100, 120, 180, 200, 240, 300, 360; T: 40, 80, 120]	Constipation, bradycardia (L)
Dihydropyridines			Ankle edema, flushing, headache, gingival hypertrophy
✓ Amlodipine (*Norvasc*)	2.5–10 (1)	[T: 2.5, 5, 10]	(L)
✓ Felodipine (*Plendil*)	2.5–20 (1)	[T: 2.5, 5, 10]	(L)
✓ Isradipine (*DynaCirc*) ✓ Sustained release (*DynaCirc CR*)	5–20 (2) 5–20 (1)	[T: 2.5, 5] [T: 5, 10]	(L)
✓ Nicardipine (*Cardene*) ✓ Sustained release (*Cardene SR*)	60–120 (3) 60–120 (2)	[C: 20, 30] [T: 30, 45, 60]	(L) (L)
✓ Nifedipine SR (*Adalat CC, Procardia XL*)	30–120 (1)	[T: 30, 60, 90]	(L)

Note: Listing of side effects is not exhaustive, and side effects are for the class of drugs except where noted for individual drugs. ✓ = preferred antihypertensive agent for treating older persons; ♥ = useful in treating heart failure.

(*continues*)

Table 16. Oral Antihypertensive Agents (cont.)			
Class, Drug	Geriatric Dose Range, total mg/d (times/d)	Formulations	Comments (Metabolism, Excretion)
✓ Nisoldipine (*Sular*)	20–60 (1)	[T: 10, 20, 30, 40]	(L)
ACE Inhibitors			Cough (common), angioedema (rare), hyperkalemia, rash, loss of taste, leukopenia
✓ ♥ Benazepril (*Lotensin*)	2.5–40 (1–2)	[T: 5, 10, 20, 40]	(L, K)
✓ ♥ Captopril (*Capoten*)	12.5–150 (2–3)	[T: 12.5, 25, 50, 100]	(L, K)
✓ ♥ Enalapril (*Vasotec*)	2.5–40 (1–2)	[T: 2.5, 5, 10, 20]	(L, K)
✓ ♥ Fosinopril (*Monopril*)	5–40 (1–2)	[T: 10, 20]	(L, K)
✓ ♥ Lisinopril (*Prinivil, Zestril*)	2.5–40 (1)	[T: 2.5, 5, 10, 20, 40]	(K)
✓ ♥ Moexipril (*Univasc*)	3.75–15 (2)	[T: 7.5, 15]	(L, K)
✓ ♥ Perindopril (*Aceon*)	4–8 (1–2)	[T: 2, 4, 8]	(L, K)
✓ ♥ Quinapril (*Accupril*)	5–80 (1–2)	[T: 5, 10, 20, 40]	(L, K)
✓ ♥ Ramipril (*Altace*)	1.25–20 (1–2)	[T: 1.25, 2.5, 5, 10]	(L, K)
✓ ♥ Trandolapril (*Mavik*)	1–4 (1)	[T: 1, 2, 4]	(L, K)
Angiotensin II Receptor Blockers (ARBs)			Angioedema (very rare), hyperkalemia
✓ ♥ Candesartan (*Atacand*)	4–32 (1)	[T: 4, 8, 16, 32]	(K)
✓ ♥ Irbesartan (*Avapro*)	75–300 (1)	[T: 75, 150, 300]	(L)
✓ ♥ Losartan (*Cozaar*)	12.5–100 (1–2)	[T: 25, 50]	(L, K)
✓ ♥ Telmisartan (*Micardis*)	20–80 (1)	[T: 20, 40, 80]	(L)
✓ ♥ Valsartan (*Diovan*)	40–320 (1)	[C: 80, 160]	(L, K)

Note: Listing of side effects is not exhaustive, and side effects are for the class of drugs except where noted for individual drugs. ✓ = preferred antihypertensive agent for treating older persons; ♥ = useful in treating heart failure.
Source: Data in part from JNC-VI: the sixth report of the Joint National Committee on Prevention, Detection, Evaluation, and Treatment of High Blood Pressure. *Arch Intern Med.* 1997;157:2413-2446.

Table 17. Choosing Antihypertensive Therapy on the Basis of Coexisting Conditions

Condition	Appropriate For Use	Avoid or Contraindicated
Angina	β, D, non-D	
Atrial tachycardia and fibrillation	β, non-D	
Bronchospasm		β, αβ
CHF	ACEI, ARB, β, αβ, L	D, non-D*
Depression		β
Diabetes mellitus	ACEI, β, T†	T†
Dyslipidemia		β, T‡
Essential tremor	β	
Hyperthyroidism	β	
MI	β, ACEI	non-D
Osteoporosis	T	
Prostatism (BPH)	α	
Renal insufficiency	ACEI§	
Urge UI	D, non-D	L, T

Note: α = α-blocker; β = β-blocker; αβ = combined α- and β-blocker; ACEI = ACE inhibitor; ARB = angiotensin receptor blocker; D = dihydropyridine calcium antagonist; non-D = nondihydropyridine calcium antagonist; L = loop diuretic; T = thiazide diuretic.
* May be beneficial in CHF caused by diastolic dysfunction.
† Low-dose diuretics are probably beneficial in type 2 diabetes; high-dose diuretics are relatively contraindicated in types 1 and 2.
‡ Low-dose diuretics have a minimal effect on lipids.
§ Use with great caution in renovascular disease.

Table 18. Antihypertensive Combinations

Drug	Trade Name
β-Adrenergic Blockers and Diuretics	
Atenolol, 50 or 100 mg *with* chlorthalidone, 25 mg	*Tenoretic*
Bisoprolol fumarate, 2.5, 5, or 10 mg *with* hydrochlorothiazide, 6.25 mg	*Ziac*
Metoprolol tartrate, 50 or 100 mg *with* hydrochlorothiazide, 25 or 50 mg	*Lopressor HCT*
Nadolol, 40 or 80 mg *with* bendroflumethiazide, 5 mg	*Corzide*
Propranolol hydrochloride, 40 or 80 mg *with* hydrochlorothiazide, 25 mg	*Inderide*
Propranolol hydrochloride (extended release), 80, 120, or 160 mg *with* hydrochlorothiazide, 50	*Inderide LA*
Timolol maleate, 10 mg *with* hydrochlorothiazide, 25 mg	*Timolide*
ACE Inhibitors and Diuretics	
Benazepril hydrochloride, 5, 10, or 20 mg *with* hydrochlorothiazide, 6.25, 12.5, or 25 mg	*Lotensin HTC*
Captopril, 25 or 50 mg *with* hydrochlorothiazide, 15 or 25 mg	*Capozide*
Enalapril maleate, 5 or 10 mg *with* hydrochlorothiazide, 12.5 or 25 mg	*Vaseretic*
Fosinopril, 10 or 20 mg *with* hydrochlorothiazide, 12.5 mg	*Monopril HCT*
Lisinopril, 10 or 20 mg *with* hydrochlorothiazide, 12.5 or 25 mg	*Prinzide, Zestoretic*
Moexipril, 7.5 or 15 mg *with* hydrochlorothiazide, 12.5 or 25 mg	*Uniretic*
Angiotensin II Receptor Blockers and Diuretics	
Candesartan, 16, 32 mg *with* hydrochlorothiazide, 12.5 mg	*Atacand-HCT*
Losartan potassium, 50 or 100 mg *with* hydrochlorothiazide, 12.5 or 25 mg	*Hyzaar*
Irbesartan, 150 or 300 mg *with* hydrochlorothiazide, 12.5 mg	*Avalide*
Telmisartan, 40, 80 mg *with* hydrochlorothiazide, 12.5 mg	*Micardis-HCT*
Valsartan, 80 mg *with* hydrochlorothiazide, 12.5 mg	*Diovan-HCT*

(continues)

Table 18. Antihypertensive Combinations (cont.)	
Drug	**Trade Name**
Calcium Antagonists and ACE Inhibitors	
Amlodipine besylate, 2.5 or 5 mg *with* benazepril hydrochloride, 10 or 20 mg	*Lotrel*
Diltiazem hydrochloride, 180 mg *with* enalapril maleate, 5 mg	*Teczem*
Felodipine, 5 mg *with* enalapril maleate, 5 mg	*Lexxel*
Verapamil hydrochloride (extended release), 180 or 240 mg *with* trandolapril, 1, 2, or 4 mg	*Tarka*
Other Combinations	
Amiloride hydrochloride, 5 mg *with* hydrochlorothiazide, 50 mg	*Moduretic*
Clonidine hydrochloride, 0.1, 0.2, or 0.3 mg *with* chlorthalidone, 15 mg	*Combipres*
Hydralazine hydrochloride, 25, 50, or 100 mg *with* hydrochlorothiazide, 25 or 50 mg	*Apresazide*
Guanethidine monosulfate, 10 mg *with* hydrochlorothiazide, 25 mg	*Esimil*
Methyldopa, 250 mg *with* chlorothiazide, 150 or 250 mg	*Aldoclor*
Methyldopa, 250 or 500 mg *with* hydrochlorothiazide, 15, 25, 30, or 50 mg	*Aldoril*
Prazosin hydrochloride, 1, 2, or 5 mg *with* polythiazide, 0.5 mg	*Minizide*
Reserpine, 0.125 or 0.25 mg *with* chlorothiazide, 250 or 500 mg	*Diupres*
Reserpine, 0.125 or 0.25 mg *with* chlorthalidone, 25 or 500 mg	*Demi-Regroton*
Reserpine, 0.10 mg *with* hydralazine hydrochloride, 25 mg *with* hydrochlorothiazide, 15 mg	*Ser-Ap-Es*
Reserpine, 0.125 mg *with* hydrochlorothiazide, 25 or 50 mg	*Hydropres*
Spironolactone, 25 or 50 mg *with* hydrochlorothiazide, 25 or 50 mg	*Aldactazide*
Triamterene, 37.5, 50, or 75 mg *with* hydrochlorothiazide, 25 or 50 mg	*Dyazide, Maxzide*

Source: JNC-VI: the sixth report of the Joint National Committee on Prevention, Detection, Evaluation, and Treatment of High Blood Pressure. *Arch Intern Med.* 1997;157:2427.

ATRIAL FIBRILLATION
Evaluation and Assessment
Causes:
• Cardiac disease: Cardiac surgery, cardiomyopathy, CHF, hypertensive heart disease, ischemic disease, pericarditis, valvular disease
• Noncardiac disease: Alcoholism, chronic pulmonary disease, infections, pulmonary emboli, thyrotoxicosis
• Standard testing: ECG, CXR, CBC, electrolytes, creatinine, BUN, TSH, echocardiogram

Management
• Correct precipitating cause(s).
• Acute-onset:
- D/C cardioversion if compromised cardiac output or angina
- If hemodynamically stable with rapid ventricular response (> 100 beats/min), lower ventricular rate medically: Options include β-blockers (eg, atenolol [*Tenormin*] 5 mg IV over 5 min, may repeat in 10 min [0.5 mg/mL], followed by 25–100 mg po qd [T: 25, 50, 100]); or calcium channel blockers (eg, diltiazem [*Cardizem injectable*] 20 mg IV bolus, giving 25 mg IV 15 min later if necessary, with a maintenance infusion of 5–15 mg/h, followed by 120–360 mg po qd of long-acting preparation [*Cardizem CD, Dilacor XR*; T: 120, 180, 240, 300, 360]. Although it works more slowly for rate control, digoxin [*Lanoxin*] is another option: 0.25 mg IV q 6 h up to 0.75 mg [0.05 mg/mL], followed by 0.125–0.25 mg po qd [T: 0.125, 0.25].

- If electric cardioversion or lowering of ventricular rate has not converted patient to sinus rhythm, begin anticoagulation with IV unfractionated heparin (see **Table 11**) followed by oral warfarin (see p 14); seek cardiology consultation for possible electric or pharmacologic cardioversion.
- Chronic AF:
- Anticoagulate (see **Table 9**) if there are no contraindications.
- If anticoagulation is contraindicated, begin aspirin 325 mg po qd.
- If electric cardioversion has not been tried in the past, seek cardiology consultation for possible cardioversion.
- Rate control (goal < 80/min averaged over 1 h) can be achieved with oral β-blockers, calcium channel blockers, or digoxin (see above for examples and dosages).

AORTIC STENOSIS (AS)
Evaluation and Assessment
- Presence of symptoms—angina, syncope, CHF (frequently diastolic dysfunction)—indicates severe disease and a life expectancy without surgery of < 2 yr.
- Echocardiography is essential in the work-up to measure aortic jet velocity (AJV) and aortic valve area (AVA). Moderate AS is indicated by an AJV of 3.0–4.0 meters/sec and by an AVA of 1.0–1.5 cm^2. Severe AS is indicated by an AJV > 4.0 meters/sec and by an AVA < 1.0 cm^2.
- For asymptomatic cases, echocardiography should be repeated annually for moderate AS and every 6–12 mo for severe AS.
- ECG and CXR should be obtained initially to look for conduction defects, LVH, and pulmonary congestion.

Treatment
- Aortic valve replacement (AVR) surgery
  - Alleviates symptoms and improves ventricular functioning.
  - In most cases, AVR should be performed promptly *after* symptoms have appeared.
  - Risks and benefits of AVR should be considered on individual basis (see pp 118–120).
- There is no effective medical treatment. Vasodilators should be avoided if possible.

PERIPHERAL ARTERIAL DISEASE

Table 19. Classes of Peripheral Arterial Disease			
Class	ABI	Symptoms	Treatment
Normal	> 0.9	None	RFM
Mild	0.8–0.9	No limitation in walking distance	RFM, AT
Moderate to severe	0.4–0.8	Walking limited by claudication	RFM, AT, CPT
Severe to critical	< 0.4	Rest pain; ischemia on exam	RFM, AT, CPT, LS

Note: ABI = ankle-brachial BP index; AT = antiplatelet therapy; CPT = claudication pain therapy, LS = limb salvage, RFM = risk factor modification.

Treatment

Risk Factor Modification:
- Low-fat diet
- Exercise: walking program
- Smoking cessation
- Lipid-lowering therapy
- BP control
- Glycemic control in diabetic patients

Antiplatelet Therapy:
- Acetylsalicylic acid (ASA) 325 mg qd
- Clopidogrel (*Plavix*) 75 mg qd [T: 75] if intolerant to ASA or aspirin failure

Claudication Pain Treatment:
- Walking program
- Drug therapy can be tried: cilostazol (*Pletal*) 100 mg bid (contraindicated in patients with CHF) 1 h before or 2 h after meals [T: 50, 100]; pentoxifylline (*Trental*) 400 mg tid [T: 400]; conventional analgesics

Limb Salvage:
- Percutaneous angioplasty
- Bypass surgery

DELIRIUM

DIAGNOSIS
Diagnostic Criteria—Adapted from *DSM-IV*
- Disturbed consciousness (ie, decreased attention, environmental awareness)
- Cognitive change (eg, memory deficit, disorientation, language disturbance), or perceptual disturbance (eg, visual illusions, hallucinations)
- Rapid onset (hours to days) and fluctuating daily course
- Evidence of a causal physical condition

Risk Factors
- Dementia greatly increases risk for delirium.
- Advanced age, comorbid physical problems, preexisting cognitive impairment

Evaluation
- Assume reversibility unless proven otherwise.
- Thoroughly review prescription and OTC medications.
- Exclude infection and other medical causes.
- Laboratory studies may include CBC, electrolytes, liver and renal function tests, serum calcium and glucose, UA, oxygen saturation, CXR, and ECG
- Confusion Assessment Method (CAM): BOTH acute onset and fluctuating course AND inattention AND EITHER disorganized thinking OR altered level of consciousness (Inouye S, *Ann Intern Med*. 1990;113:941–948).

CAUSES
Drugs
- Anticholinergics (eg, diphenhydramine), tricyclic antidepressants (eg, amitriptyline, imipramine), antipsychotics (eg, chlorpromazine, thioridazine)
- Anti-inflammatory agents, including prednisone
- Benzodiazepines or alcohol—acute toxicity or withdrawal
- Cardiovascular (eg, digitalis, antihypertensives)
- Diuretics
- Lithium
- GI (eg, cimetidine, ranitidine)
- Opioid analgesics (especially meperidine)

Infections
Respiratory, skin, urinary tract, and others

Metabolic Disorders
Acute blood loss, electrolyte imbalance, end-organ failure (hepatic, renal), hypo- or hyperglycemia, hypoxia

Cardiovascular
Arrhythmia, CHF, MI, shock

Neurologic
CNS infections, head trauma, seizures, stroke, subdural hematoma, TIAs, tumors

Miscellaneous
Fecal impaction, postoperative state, sleep deprivation, urinary retention

PREVENTION

Table 20. Risk Factors and Interventions to Prevent Delirium	
Targeted Risk Factor	Interventions
Cognitive impairment (MMSE total score < 20 or orientation score < 8)	Orientation board; communication to reorient surroundings
	Cognitively stimulating activities (eg, current events discussion, word games)
Sleep deprivation	Warm drink at bedtime, relaxation tapes or music, back massage, nighttime noise reduction
Immobility	Ambulation or active range-of-motion exercises
Visual impairment (< 20/70 visual acuity on binocular near-vision testing)	Visual aids (eg, glasses, magnifying lenses), adaptive equipment (eg, large illuminated telephone keypads, large-print books)
Hearing impairment (hearing < 6 of 12 whispers on whisper test)	Portable amplifying device, earwax disimpaction
Dehydration (BUN/creatinine ratio > 18)	Volume repletion (eg, encourage oral fluid intake)

Source: Table adapted from data published in Inouye SK, Bogardus ST, Charpentier PA, et al. A multicomponent intervention to prevent delirium in hospitalized older patients. *N Engl J Med.* 1999;340:669–676.

MANAGEMENT

Nonpharmacologic (See also **Table 20**)
- Identify and remove or treat underlying cause
- Provide general supportive measures:
  - Keep patient in quiet, well-lit room (eg, night lights)
  - Avoid excessive noise, stimulation
  - Encourage familiar faces (family members) at bedside for reassurance
  - Provide orientation (eg, calendar, clock)
  - Correct sensory impairment (eg, vision, hearing)
  - Communicate in succinct, direct style
  - Use a sitter
  - Use physical restraints only as last resort to maintain patient safety (eg, prevent patient from pulling out tubes, catheters)

Pharmacologic
- For acute agitation or aggression accompanying delirium, use a high-potency antipsychotic such as haloperidol (*Haldol*) 0.5–2 mg po [T: 0.5, 1, 2, 5, 10, 20; S: 2 mg/mL] or IV or IM (twice as potent as po). May also be given as slow IV push; titrate upward as needed. Reevaluate every 30 min. Observe for development of EPS. Avoid low-potency antipsychotics such as chlorpromazine (*Thorazine*) or thioridazine (*Mellaril*) because of their anticholinergic and arrythmogenic properties (torsade de pointes). If patient is able to take drugs po, consider low dose of atypical antipsychotic (see **Table 68**).
- If delirium is secondary to alcohol or benzodiazepine withdrawal, use a benzodiazepine such as lorazepam (*Ativan*) in doses of 0.5–2 mg every 4–6 h. Since these agents themselves may cause delirium, gradual withdrawal and discontinuation are desirable. If delirium is secondary to alcohol, also use thiamine 100 mg qd (po, IM, or IV).

DEMENTIA

DEMENTIA SYNDROME
Definition
Acquired decline in memory and in at least one other cognitive function
(eg, language, visual spatial, executive) sufficient to affect daily life in an alert person.

Estimated Frequencies of Dementia Causes
• AD: 60% to 70%
• Other progressive disorders: 15% to 30% (eg, vascular, Lewy body)
• Completely reversible dementia (eg, drug toxicity, metabolic changes, thyroid
  disease, subdural hematoma, normal-pressure hydrocephalus): 2% to 5%

DIAGNOSIS OF AD
• Dementia syndrome
• Gradual onset and continuing decline
• Not due to another physical, neurologic, or psychiatric condition or to medications
• Deficits not occurring exclusively during delirium

STAGES OF AD
Mild Cognitive Impairment   (preclinical)   MMSE: 26–30
- Delayed paragraph recall
- Cognition otherwise intact
- No functional impairment
- Mild construction, language, or executive dysfunction

Early, Mild Impairment   (yr 1–3 from onset of symptoms)   MMSE: 22–28
- Disorientation for date
- Naming difficulties (anomia)
- Recent recall problems
- Mild difficulty copying figures
- Decreased insight
- Social withdrawal
- Irritability, mood change
- Problems managing finances

Middle, Moderate Impairment   (yr 2–8)   MMSE: 10–21
- Disoriented to date, place
- Comprehension difficulties (aphasia)
- Impaired new learning
- Getting lost in familiar areas
- Impaired calculating skills
- Delusions, agitation, aggression
- Not cooking, shopping, banking
- Restless, anxious, depressed
- Problems with dressing, grooming

Late, Severe Impairment   (yr 6–12)   MMSE: 0–9
- Nearly unintelligible verbal output
- Remote memory gone
- Unable to copy or write
- No longer grooming or dressing
- Incontinent
- Motor or verbal agitation

NONCOGNITIVE SYMPTOMS

Psychotic Symptoms (eg, Delusions, Hallucinations)
- Occur in about one third of AD patients
- Delusions may be paranoid (eg, people stealing things, spouse unfaithful)
- Hallucinations more commonly visual

Depressive Symptoms
- Occur in up to 40% of AD patients; may herald onset of AD
- May cause acceleration of decline if untreated
- Need to suspect if patient stops eating or withdraws

Agitation or Aggression
- Occurs in up to 80% of patients with AD
- A leading cause of nursing-home admission
- Consider superimposed delirium or pain as a trigger

RISK AND PROTECTIVE FACTORS FOR AD

Definite Risks	Possible Risks	Possible Protections
Age	Other genes	Estrogen
Family history	Head trauma	NSAIDs
Down syndrome	Lower educational level	Antioxidants
APOE-E4	Depression	

Clinical Features Distinguishing AD and Other Types of Dementia
- AD: Memory, language, visuospatial disturbances, indifference, delusions, agitation
- Frontotemporal dementia: Personality change, executive dysfunction, hyperorality, relative preservation of visuospatial skills
- Lewy body dementia: visual hallucinations, delusions, extrapyramidal symptoms, fluctuating mental status, sensitivity to antipsychotic medications

EVALUATION

Although completely reversible (eg, drug toxicity) dementia is rare, identifying and treating secondary physical conditions may improve function.
- History: Obtain from family or other informant
- Physical and neurologic examination
- Assess functional status
- Evaluate mental status (eg, Mini-Cog, see p 161; number of animals named in 1 min; MMSE; GDS, p 165)

Laboratory Testing
CBC, TSH, B_{12}, serum calcium, liver and renal function tests, electrolytes, serologic test for syphilis; at this time genetic testing and commercial "Alzheimer blood tests" are not recommended for clinical use.

Neuroimaging
The likelihood of detecting structural lesions is increased with:
- Onset age < 60
- Focal (unexplained) neurologic signs or symptoms

- Abrupt onset or rapid decline (weeks to months)
- Predisposing conditions (eg, metastatic cancer or anticoagulants)

Neuroimaging may detect the 5% of patients with clinically significant structural lesions that would otherwise be missed.

TREATMENT
Primary goals of treatment are to improve quality of life and maximize functional performance by enhancing cognition, mood, and behavior.

General Treatment Principles
- Identify and treat comorbid physical illnesses (eg, hypertension, diabetes mellitus)
- Set realistic goals
- Limit prn psychotropic medication use
- Specify and quantify target behaviors
- Maximize and maintain functioning

Nonpharmacologic Approaches
To improve function:
- Behavior modification, scheduled toileting, and prompted toileting (see p 152) for UI
- Graded assistance (as little help as possible to perform ADLs), practice, and positive reinforcement to increase independence

For problem behaviors:
- Music during meals, bathing
- Walking or light exercise
- Simulate family presence with video or audio tapes
- Pet therapy
- Speak at patient's comprehension level
- Bright light, white noise

Pharmacologic Treatment of Cognitive Dysfunction in AD
Patients with a diagnosis of mild or moderate AD should receive a cholinesterase inhibitor that will increase level of acetylcholine in brain (**Table 21**) (demonstrated benefit for cognition, mood, behavioral symptoms, and daily function). Consider the antioxidant vitamin E at 1000 IU bid (shown to delay functional decline thought to occur from oxidative stress). Controlled data show benefits of cholinergic drugs for 1 yr and open trials demonstrate benefit for 3 yr. Only 25% of patients taking cholinesterase inhibitors show clinical improvement but 80% have less rapid decline. Initial studies show benefits of these drugs for patients with Lewy body dementia and dementia with vascular risk factors. Prolonged cholinergic therapy may delay nursing-home placement. To evaluate response or stabilize:
- Elicit caregiver observations of patient's behavior (alertness, initiative) and follow functional status (ADLs and IADLs).
- Follow cognitive status (eg, improved or stabilized) by caregiver's report or serial ratings of cognition (eg, Mini-Cog, see p 161; MMSE).
- Ginkgo biloba is not generally recommended because clinical trial results are not yet definitive, and preparations vary since such nutriceuticals are not FDA regulated.

Table 21. Cholinesterase Inhibitors*

Drug	Formulations	Dosing
Donepezil (Aricept)	[T: 5, 10]	Start at 5 mg qd, increase to 10 mg qd after 1 mo
Galantamine (Reminyl)	[T: 4, 8, 12; S: 4 mg/mL]	Start at 4 mg bid, increase to 8 mg bid after 4 wk; recommended dose 16–24 mg/d
Rivastigmine (Exelon)	[T: 1.5, 3, 4.5, 6]	Start at 1.5 mg bid and gradually titrate up to 6 mg bid as tolerated; retitrate if drug is stopped

* Side effects increase with higher dosing. Continue if improvement or stabilization occurs; stopping drugs can lead to rapid decline. Possible side effects include nausea, vomiting, diarrhea, dyspepsia, anorexia, weight loss, leg cramps, bradycardia, and agitation.

Treatment of Agitation

Table 22. Agitation Treatment Guidelines

Symptom	Drug*	Dosage	Formulations
Agitation in context of nonacute psychosis	Risperidone (Risperdal)	0.25–1.5 mg/d	[T: 0.25, 0.5, 1, 2, 3, 4; S: 1 mg/mL]
	Olanzapine (Zyprexa)	2.5–10 mg/d	[T: 2.5, 5, 7.5, 10, 15, 20]
	Quetiapine (Seroquel)	25–400 mg/d	[T: 25, 100, 200, 300]
	Thiothixene (Navane)	2–4 mg/d**	[C: 1, 2, 5, 10, 20]
Acute psychosis agitation if IM or IV is needed	Droperidol (Inapsine)	0.5–2 mg/d**	[IM, IV: 2.5 mg/mL]
	Haloperidol (Haldol)	0.5–2 mg/d**	[T: 0.5, 1, 2, 5, 10, 20; S: 2 mg/mL; Inj: 5 mg/mL]
Agitation in context of depression	SSRI, eg, citalopram (Celexa)	10–30 mg/d	[T: 20, 40; L: 2mg/mL]
Anxiety, mild to moderate irritability	Trazodone (Desyrel)	50–100 mg/d†	[T: 50, 100, 150, 300]
	Buspirone (BuSpar)	30–60 mg/d‡	[T: 5, 10, 15, 30]
As a possible second-line treatment for significant agitation or aggression	Divalproex sodium (Depakote)	500–1500 mg/d§	[T: 125, 250, 500; syrup 250 mg/mL, sprinkles]
	Carbamazepine (Tegretol)	300–600 mg/d§§	[T: 100, 200; suspension 100/5 mL]
Sexual aggression, impulse-control symptoms in men	Estrogen (Premarin) or medroxyprogesterone (Depo-Provera)	0.625–1.25 mg/d 100 mg IM /wk	[T: 0.3, 0.625, 0.9, 1.25, 2.5] [Inj: 100, 150, 400 mg/mL]

*All metabolized by the liver.
** May need to give higher doses in emergency situations; should be used for only short periods of time.
† Small divided daytime dosage and larger bedtime dosage; watch for sedation and orthostasis.
‡ Can be given bid; 2–4 wk for adequate trial.
§ Can monitor serum levels; usually well tolerated; check CBC, platelets for agranulocytosis, thrombocytopenia risk in older patients.
§§ Monitor serum levels; periodic CBCs, platelet counts secondary to agranulocytosis risk. Beware of drug-drug interactions.

CAREGIVER ISSUES

- Over 50% develop depression.
- Physical illness, isolation, anxiety, and burnout are common.
- Intensive education and support of caregivers may delay institutionalization.
- Adult day care for patients and respite services may help.
- Alzheimer's Association offers support, education; chapters are located in major cities throughout US. (See p 230 for telephone, Web site.)
- Family Caregiver Alliance offers support, education, information for caregivers. (See p 230 for telephone, Web site.)

REPORT OF THE QUALITY STANDARDS SUBCOMMITTEE OF THE AAN

Doody RS, Stevens JC, Beck C, et al. Practice parameter: management of dementia (an evidence-based review): report of the Quality Standards Subcommittee of the American Academy of Neurology. *Neurology* 2001; 56(9):1154–1166.

DEPRESSION

EVALUATION AND ASSESSMENT

Recognizing and diagnosing late-life depression can be difficult. Older patients may complain of lack of energy or other somatic symptoms, attribute symptoms to old age or other physical conditions, or fail to mention them to a health care professional.

Medical Evaluation

TSH, B$_{12}$, calcium, LFTs, renal function tests, electrolytes, UA, CBC

DSM-IV Criteria for Major Depressive Episode (Abbreviated)

Five or more of the following symptoms have been present during the same 2-wk period and represent a change from previous functioning; at least one of the symptoms is either (1) depressed mood or (2) loss of interest or pleasure.

- Depressed mood
- Loss of interest or pleasure in activities
- Significant weight loss or gain (not intentional), or decrease or increase in appetite
- Insomnia or hypersomnia
- Psychomotor agitation or retardation
- Fatigue or loss of energy
- Feelings of worthlessness or excessive or inappropriate guilt
- Diminished ability to think or concentrate, or indecisiveness
- Recurrent thoughts of death, suicidal ideation, attempt, or plan

The *DSM-IV* criteria are not specific for older adults; cognitive symptoms may be more prominent. The GDS is useful for screening and monitoring (see p 165).

MANAGEMENT

Treatment should be individualized on the basis of history, past response, and severity of illness as well as concurrent illnesses. Treatments may be combined.

Nonpharmacologic

For mild to moderate depression or in combination with pharmacotherapy: cognitive-behavioral therapy, interpersonal therapy, problem-solving therapy.

Pharmacologic

For mild, moderate or severe depression: the duration of therapy should be at least 6–12 mo following remission for patients experiencing their first depressive episode. Most older patients with a history of major depression require lifelong antidepressant therapy.

42

Choosing an Antidepressant (see Table 23 and Table 24)

Consider an SSRI: As first-line choice for most older patients, especially:

- Patients with heart conduction defects or ischemic heart disease
- Patients with prostatic hyperplasia
- Patients with uncontrolled glaucoma

Consider Venlafaxine, Mirtazapine, or Bupropion: As second-line choice

Consider Nortriptyline or Desipramine:

- As a third-line treatment for severe melancholic depression
- For patients with urge incontinence, but use tolterodine (*Detrol*) and an SSRI if avoidance of central anticholinergic effects of a TCA is important (see **Table 78**)

Table 23. Antidepressants Used for Older Adults				
Class, Drug	Initial Dosage	Usual Dosage	Formulations	Comments (Metabolism, Excretion)
Selective Serotonin-Reuptake Inhibitors				
Citalopram (*Celexa*)	10–20 mg qam	20–30 mg/d	[T: 20, 40, 60]	Class side effects (EPS, hyponatremia) (L, K [10%])
Fluoxetine (*Prozac*)	5 mg qam	5–60 mg/d	[T: 10; C: 10, 20, 40; S: 20 mg/5 mL C: SR 190 (weekly dose)]	Long half-lives of parent and active metabolite may allow for less frequent dosing; CYP2D6, -2C9, -3A4 inhibitor (L)
Fluvoxamine (*Luvox*)	25 mg qhs	100–300 mg/d	[T: 25, 50, 100]	Not approved as an antidepressant in US ; CYP1A2, -3A4 inhibitor (L)
Paroxetine (*Paxil*)	5 mg	10–40 mg/d	[T: 10, 20, 30, 40]	Helpful if anxiety symptoms are prominent ; CYP2D6 inhibitor (L)
Sertraline (*Zoloft*)	25 mg qam	50–200 mg/d	[T: 25, 50, 100]	(L)
Other				
Bupropion (*Wellbutrin, Zyban*)	37.5–50 mg bid 100 mg (SR) qd or bid	75–150 mg bid 100–150 mg (SR) bid	[T: 75, 100; SR 100, 150]	Consider for SSRI, TCA nonresponders; safe in CHF; may be stimulating; can lower seizure threshold (L)
Methylphenidate (*Ritalin*)	2.5–5 mg at 7 AM and noon	5–10 mg at 7 AM and noon	[T: 5, 10, 20]	Short-term treatment of depression or apathy in physically ill elderly; used as an adjunct (L)
Mirtazapine (*Remeron*)	15 mg qhs	15–45 mg/d	[T: 15, 30, 45]	May increase appetite; sedating; oral disintegrating tablet (SolTab) available (L)

(continues)

Table 23. Antidepressants Used for Older Adults (cont.)				
Class, Drug	Initial Dosage	Usual Dosage	Formulations	Comments (Metabolism, Excretion)
Nefazodone (*Serzone*)	50 mg bid	200–400 mg/d	[T: 50, 100, 150, 200, 250]	May help insomnia; sedating in some patients; CYP3A4 inhibition (L)
Trazodone (*Desyrel*)	25 mg qhs	75–600 mg/d	[T: 50, 100, 150, 300]	Sedation may limit dose; may be used as a hypnotic; ventricular irritability; priapism in men (L)
Venlafaxine (*Effexor*)	25–50 mg bid	75–225 mg/d	[T: 25, 37.5, 50, 75, 100]	Low anticholinergic activity; minimal sedation and hypotension; may increase BP; may be useful when somatic pain present (L)
(*Effexor XR*)	75 mg qam	75–225 mg/d	[C: 37.5, 75, 150]	EPS, hyponatremia
Tricyclic Antidepressants				
Desipramine (*Norpramin*)	10–25 mg qhs	50–150 mg/d	[T: 10, 25, 50, 75, 100, 150]	Therapeutic serum level > 115 ng/mL (L)
Nortriptyline (*Aventyl, Pamelor*)	10–25 mg qhs	75–150 mg/d	[C: 10, 25, 50, 75; S: 10 mg/5 mL]	Therapeutic window (50–150 ng/mL) (L)
Monoamine Oxidase Inhibitors				
Isocarboxazid (*Marplan*)	10 mg bid–tid	10 mg tid	[T: 10]	Hypotension; drug, food interactions (K, L)
Phenelzine (*Nardil*)	15 mg qd	15–60 mg/d	[T: 15]	Hypotension; drug, food interactions (L, K)
Tranylcypromine (*Parnate*)	10 mg bid	20–40 mg/d	[T: 10]	Hypotension; drug, food interactions (L)

Table 24. Antidepressants to Avoid in Older Adults			
Class, Drug	Usual Dosage	Formulations	Comments (Metabolism, Excretion)
Heterocyclic Antidepressants			
Amitriptyline (eg, *Elavil*)	25–150 mg/d	[T: 10, 25, 50, 75, 100, 150; Inj: 10 mg/mL]	Anticholinergic, sedating, hypotension (L)
Amoxapine (*Asendin*)	50–150 mg/d	[T: 25, 50, 100, 150]	See amitriptyline; also associated with extrapyramidal effects, tardive dyskinesia, and neuroleptic malignant syndrome (L)

Table 24. Antidepressants to Avoid in Older Adults (cont.)

Class, Drug	Usual Dosage	Formu-lations	Comments (Metabolism, Excretion)
Clomipramine (*Anafranil*)	100–250 mg/d	[C: 25, 50, 75]	Used to treat OCD (L)
Doxepin (eg, *Sinequan*)	25–150 mg/d	[C: 10, 25, 50, 75, 100, 150; S: 10 mg/mL]	See amitriptyline (L)
Imipramine (eg, *Tofranil*)	50–150 mg/d	[C: as pamoate 75, 100, 125, 150; Inj; T: as hydrochloride 10, 25, 50]	See amitriptyline (L)
Maprotiline (*Ludiomil*)	50–75 mg/d	[T: 25, 50, 75]	Seizures and rashes (L)
Protriptyline (*Vivactil*)	5–20 mg/d	[T: 5, 10]	Very anticholinergic; can be stimulating (L)
St. John's wort	–	–	Decreases effects of digoxin and 3A4 substrates; efficacy questioned
Trimipramine (*Surmontil*)	25–100 mg/d	[C: 25, 50, 100]	See amitriptyline (L)

Electroconvulsive Therapy
Generally safe and very effective.

Indications: Severe depression when a rapid onset of response is necessary; when depression is resistant to drug therapy; for patients who are unable to tolerate antidepressants, have previous response to ECT, have psychotic depression, severe catatonia, or depression with Parkinson's disease.

Complications: Temporary confusion, arrhythmias, aspiration, falls.

Contraindications:
- Increased intracranial pressure
- Intracranial tumor
- MI within 3 mo (relative)
- Stroke within 1 mo (relative)

Before ECT evaluation: CXR, ECG, serum electrolytes, and cardiac examination. Additional tests (eg, stress test, neuroimaging, EEG) are used selectively.

DERMATOLOGIC CONDITIONS

COMMON DERMATOLOGIC CONDITIONS

Table 25. Dermatologic Conditions Common in Elderly Persons

Condition	Areas Affected	Description	Risk Factors, Comments
Candidiasis	Body folds	Erythema, pustules, or cheesy, whitish matter, satellite lesions	Intertrigo, diabetes mellitus, poor hygiene
Treatment: See intertrigo, below; antifungal powders			
Intertrigo	Any place 2 skin surfaces rest against one another (eg, under the breasts)	Moist, erythematous with local superficial skin loss; satellite lesions due to candida	Obesity, diabetes mellitus, immobility
Treatment: Keep area dry; topical antifungals (see below), absorbent powder, 1% hydrocortisone or 0.1% triamcinolone cream bid × 1 or 2 d if inflamed			
Neurodermatitis	Any skin surfaces	Generalized, localized itching	Irritants, xerosis, scabies, allergic contact dermatitis
Treatment: Mid- to higher-potency topical corticosteroids; exclude other causes			
Onychomycosis	Nails	Thickening and discoloration	
Treatment: Itraconazole (*Sporanox*)—toenails: 200 mg po qd × 3 mo or 400 mg po qd × 1 wk/mo × 3–4 mo; fingernails: 400 mg po qd × 1 wk/mo × 3–4 mo (L); fluconazole (*Diflucan*)—toenails: 150 or 300 mg po/wk × 6–12 mo; fingernails: 150 or 300 mg po/wk × 3–6 mo (L); terbinafine (*Lamisil*)—toenails: 250 mg po qd × 12 wk; fingernails: 250 mg qd × 6 wk. Obtain nail specimens for laboratory culturing to confirm diagnosis before prescribing itraconazol or terbinafine			
Psoriasis	All skin areas, nails (pitting)	Well-defined, erythematous plaques covered with silver scales; severity varies	All ages, can be drug-induced
Treatment: Topical corticosteroids, UV light, PUVA, methotrexate, cyclosporin, etretinate, sulfasalazine; anthralin preparations and tar + 1% to 4% salicylic acid; calcipotriene for nonfacial areas			
Rosacea	Face	Vascular & follicular dilation; mild to moderate	
Treatment: Topical metronidazole gel 0.75% bid; oral doxycycline 100 mg qd			
Scabies	Interdigital webs, flexor aspects of wrists, axillary, umbilicus, nipples, genitals	Burrows, erythematous papules or nodules, dry or scaly skin, pruritus	Can result in epidemics
Treatment: Apply topical products from head to toe: Permethrin (*Elimite*) 5% cream 8–14 h, remove; crotamiton (*Eurax*) 10% cream × 24 h, repeat, then cleansing bath in 48 h; or 1% lindane (*K-well, Scabene*) cream × 8–12 h, remove; oatmeal baths, topical corticosteroids or emollient creams for symptom relief; ivermectin (*Mectizan, Stromectol*) 200 μg/kg orally; may repeat once in 1 or 2 wk [T: 6]			

Table 25. Dermatologic Conditions Common in Elderly Persons (cont.)

Condition	Areas Affected	Description	Risk Factors, Comments
Seborrheic dermatitis	Nasal labial folds, eyebrows, hairline, sideburns, posterior auriculare and midchest	Greasy, yellow scales with or without erythematous base; common in Parkinson's disease and in debilitated patients	All age groups

Treatment: Hydrocortisone 1% cream bid or triamcinolone 0.1% ointment bid × 2 wk; scalp: shampoo (selenium sulfide, zinc, or tar); ketoconazole 2% cream for severe conditions when infection from *Pityrosporum orbiculare* is suspected

Skin maceration	Any area constantly in contact with moisture, covered with occlusive dressing or bandage; skin folds, groin, buttocks	Erythema; abraded, excoriated skin; blisters; white and silver patches	Urinary or fecal incontinence, wound and fistula drainage, leakage around ostomy or GI tube sites

Treatment: Eliminate cause of moisture: toileting program for incontinence; condom catheter; indwelling catheter (reserve for most intractable conditions); fecal incontinence collector. Protect skin from moisture: clean gently with mild soap after each incontinent episode; apply moisture barrier (eg, *Vaseline, Proshield, Smooth and Cool, Calmoseptene*) to repel moisture; use disposable briefs that wick moisture from the skin; use linen incontinence pads when disposable briefs accentuate perineal dermatitis.

Urticaria: Hives	Skin surface	Uniform, red edematous plaques surrounded by white halos	—

Treatment: Identify cause, oral H$_1$ antihistamines (see **Table 70**), oral glucocorticoids (eg, prednisone 40 mg qd), oral H$_2$ antihistamines, or doxepin for refractory cases.

Urticaria: Angioedema	Lips, eyelids, tongue, larynx, GI tract	Larger, deeper than hives	Allergies (medications, nuts)

Treatment: Oral H$_1$ antihistamines (see **Table 70**), oral glucocorticoids. Severe reactions: SC epinephrine 0.3 mL of a 1:1000 dilution (*EpiPen*)

Urticaria: Cholinergic	Skin surface	Round, red papular wheals	Exercise, heat, stress

Treatment: Oral H$_1$ antihistamines (see **Table 70**) 1 h before exercise. Hot shower may relieve itching.

Xerosis	All skin surfaces	Dull, rough, flaky, cracked; nummular	Low humidity, winter, aging

Treatment: ↑ Humidity, apply emollient ointment (eg, *Aquaphor*) or cream (eg, *Eucerin*) immediately after bathing; oatmeal baths; hydrocortisone 1% ointment; avoid excess bathing and bath oils (falls)

Topical Antifungals

- Amphotericin B (*Fungizone*) [3% cream, lotion, or ointment]
- Clotrimazole (*Lotrimin, Mycelex*) [1% cream, lotion, solution]
- Econazole nitrate (*Spectazole*) [1% cream]
- Ketoconazole (*Nizoral*) [2% cream or shampoo]
- Miconazole (eg, *Monistat-Derm*) [2% cream, lotion, powder, spray, tincture]
- Nystatin (*Mycostatin, Nilstat, Nystex*) [100,000 units/g cream, ointment, powder]
- Ternafine (*Lamisil*–OTC) [1% cream, gel]

Oral Antifungals

- Fluconazole (*Diflucan*) [T: 50, 100, 150, 200; S: 10, 40 mg/mL]
- Itraconazole (*Sporonax*) [C: 100; S: 100 mg/mL]
- Terbinafine (*Lamisil*) [T: 250]

DERMATOLOGIC MEDICATIONS

Table 26. Topical Corticosteroids		
Name	**Strength & Formulations**	**Frequency of Application**
Lowest Potency		
Dexamethasone phosphate (*Decaderm*)	0.1% cream	qd–qid
Hydrocortisone acetate (*Hytone*)	0.25%, 0.5%, 1%, 2.5% cream, ointment	tid–qid
Low Potency		
Alclometasone dipropionate (*Aclovate*)	0.5% cream, ointment	bid–tid
Betamethasone valerate (*Valisone*)	0.1% lotion	bid–qid
Desonide (*DesOwen, Tridesilon*)	0.05% cream	bid–qid
Fluocinolone acetonide (*Synalar*)	0.025% cream, 0.01% solution	bid–qid
Triamcinolone acetonide (*Aristocort, Kenalog*)	0.1% cream, 0.025% cream, lotion, ointment	bid–tid
Mid-potency		
Betamethasone dipropionate (*Diprosone*)	0.05% lotion	bid–qid
Betamethasone valerate (*Valisone*)	0.1% cream	bid–qid
Clocortolone pivalate (*Cloderm*)	0.1% cream	qd–qid
Desoximetasone (*Topicort*)	0.5% cream	bid
Fluocinolone acetonide (*Synalar*)	0.025% cream, ointment	bid–qid
Flurandrenolide (*Cordran*)	0.05% cream, ointment	qd–bid
Fluticasone propionate (*Cutivate*)	0.05% cream	bid
Hydrocortisone butyrate (*Locoid*)	0.1% cream	qd–bid
Hydrocortisone valerate (*Westcort*)	0.2% cream, ointment	tid–qid
Mometasone furoate (*Elocon*)	0.1% cream, lotion	qd
Triamcinolone acetonide (*Aristocort, Kenalog*)	0.1% lotion, ointment	bid–tid
High Potency		
Amcinonide (*Cyclocort*)	0.1% cream, lotion	bid–tid
Betamethasone dipropionate (*Diprosone*)	0.05% cream	bid–qid
Betamethasone valerate (*Valisone*)	0.01% ointment	bid–qid
Diflorasone diacetate (*Florone, Maxiflor*)	0.05% cream	bid–qid
Fluocinonide (*Lidex-E*)	0.05% cream	bid–qid
Fluticasone propionate (*Cutivate*)	0.005% ointment	bid
Triamcinolone acetonide (*Aristocort, Kenalog*)	0.5% ointment	bid–tid
Higher Potency		
Amcinonide (*Cyclocort*)	0.1% ointment	bid–tid
Betamethasone dipropionate (*Diprolene AF*)	0.05% augmented cream	bid–qid
Betamethasone dipropionate (*Diprosone*)	0.05% ointment	bid–qid

Table 26. Topical Corticosteroids (cont.)		
Name	Strength & Formulations	Frequency of Application
Desoximetasone (*Topicort*)	0.25% cream, ointment; 0.05% gel	bid
Diflorasone diacetate (*Florone, Maxiflor*)	0.05% ointment	bid–qid
Fluocinonide (*Lidex*)	0.05% cream, ointment, gel	bid–qid
Halcinonide (*Halog*)	0.1% cream	qd–tid
Mometasone furoate (*Elocon*)	0.1% ointment	qd
Super Potency		
Betamethasone dipropionate (*Diprolene*)	0.05% augmented cream, ointment	bid–qid
Clobetasol propionate (*Temovate*)	0.05% cream, ointment	bid
Diflorasone diacetate (*Psorcon*)	0.05% optimized ointment	qd–tid
Halobetasol propionate (*Ultravate*)	0.05% cream and ointment	bid

ADRENAL INSUFFICIENCY
Pharmacologic Therapy
For corticosteroid dose equivalencies, see **Table 27**, below.

Management
Stress doses of corticosteroids for patients with severe illness, injury, or undergoing surgery: Give hydrocortisone 100 mg IV q 8 h. For less severe stress, double or triple usual oral replacement dose and taper back to baseline as quickly as possible.

Table 27. Corticosteroids					
Drug	Approx Equivalent Dose (mg)	Relative Anti-In-flammatory Potency	Relative Mineral-corticoid	Biologic Half-Life (h)	Formulations
Betamethasone (*Celestone*)	0.6–0.75	20–30	0	36–54	[T: 0.6; S: 0.6 mg/5 mL]
Cortisone (*Cortone*)	25	0.8	2	8–12	[T: 5; S: 50 mg/mL]
Dexamethasone (*Decadron, Dexone, Hexadrol*)	0.75	20–30	0	36–54	[T: 0.25, 0.5, 0.75, 1, 1.5, 2, 4; elixir: 0.5 mg/5 mL; Inj: 4 mg/mL]
Fludrocortisone (*Florinef*) *	NA	10	4	12–36	[T: 0.1]
Hydrocortisone (*Cortef, Hydrocortone*)	20	1	2	8–12	[T: 5, 10, 20; Inj: 50 mg/mL; S: 10 mg/5 mL]
Methylprednisolone (eg, *Medrol, Solu-Medrol, Depo-Medrol*)	4	5	0	18–36	[T: 2, 4, 8, 16, 24, 32; Inj: 40, 125, 500, 1000 mg]
Prednisolone (eg, *Delta-Cortef, Prelone Syrup, Pediapred*)	5	4	1	18–36	[syrup: 5, 15 mg/5 mL; S: 5 mg/5 mL]
Prednisone (*Deltasone, Liquid Pred, Meticorten, Orasone*)	5	4	1	18–36	[T: 1, 2.5, 5, 10, 20, 50; S: 5 mg/5 mL]
Triamcinolone (eg, *Aristo-cort, Kenacort, Kenalog*)	4	5	0	18–36	[T: 1, 2, 4, 8; syrup: 4 mg/5 mL]

Note: NA = not available.
*Usually given for orthostatic hypotension 0.1 mg qd–tid.

THYROID DISEASE
Pharmacologic Therapy
Hypothyroidism:
- Thyroxine (T$_4$, levothyroxine [*Eltroxin, Levo-T, Levothroid, Levoxyl, Synthroid*]). Start 25 µg and increase by 25-µg intervals every 4–6 wk [T: 25, 50, 75, 88, 100, 112, 125, 137, 150, 175, 200, 300 µg].
- Thyroxine and liothyronine (T$_3$) (*Thyrolar*). Start ¼ strength and increase [12.5/3.1 (¼ strength), 25/6.25 (½ strength), 50/12.5, 100/25, 150/37.5 µg].
- For myxedema coma: Load 400 µg IV or 100 µg q 6–8 h for 1 d; then 100 µg/d for 4 d; then start usual replacement regimen.
- To convert thyroid USP to thyroxine: 60 mg USP = 50 µg thyroxine.
- If patients are npo and must receive IV thyroxine, dose should be half usual po dose.

Hyperthyroidism:
- Radioactive iodine ablation is usual treatment of choice, but surgery or medical therapy (see below) are options.
- Propylthiouracil (PTU): Start 100 po tid, then adjust up to 200 po tid as needed [T: 50].
- Methimazole (*Tapazole*): Start 5–20 mg po tid, then adjust [T: 5, 10].
- Adjunctive therapy with β-blockers (see p 28) or calcium antagonists (see p 29) may provide symptomatic improvement.

Management and Monitoring
- In primary hypothyroidism, the goal of therapy is to maintain plasma TSH within the normal range. Further adjustments are made every 6–12 wk (12- to 25-µg increments) on basis of TSH levels until TSH is in normal range. Monitor TSH level every 6–12 mo (ATA) in patients on chronic thyroid replacement therapy. Following dose adjustment, recheck TSH in 6–12 wk.
- Amiodarone-induced hypothyroidism is rare after the first 18 mo of therapy; amiodarone-induced thyrotoxicosis can occur any time during therapy. Check TSH every few mo. Manage hypothyroidism as above. Consult endocrinologist and cardiologist if patient becomes thyrotoxic.

DIABETES MELLITUS
Definition and Classification (ADA)
Diabetes mellitus is a group of metabolic diseases characterized by hyperglycemia resulting from defects in insulin secretion, insulin action, or both.
Type 1: Caused by an absolute deficiency of insulin secretion.
Type 2: Caused by a combination of resistance to insulin action and an inadequate compensatory insulin secretory response.
Criteria for Diagnosis: One or more of the following:
- Symptoms of diabetes (eg, polyuria, polydipsia, unexplained weight loss) plus casual plasma glucose concentration ≥ 200 mg/dL
- Fasting (no caloric intake for ≥ 8 h) plasma glucose ≥ 126 mg/dL
- 2 h Plasma glucose ≥ 200 mg/dL during an oral glucose tolerance test (OGTT)
  Diagnosis should be confirmed by reevaluating on a subsequent day.
Impaired Fasting Glucose: Defined as fasting plasma glucose ≥ 110 and < 126 mg/dL

Impaired Glucose Tolerance: Abnormal casual plasma glucose concentration or response to OGTT but not meeting diagnostic criteria for diabetes

Management
Goals of Treatment (ADA): Average preprandial capillary blood glucose 80–120 mg/dL, average bedtime capillary blood glucose 100–140 mg/dL, and $HbA_{1c} < 7\%$
Nonpharmacologic Interventions:
- Individualized nutrition
- Life style (eg, exercise, alcohol and smoking cessation)
- Patient and family education for self-management
- Self-monitoring of blood glucose

Pharmacologic Interventions for Type 2: Stepped therapy:
1. Monotherapy with a 2nd-generation sulfonylurea agent, α-glucosidase inhibitor, metformin, or thiazolidinedione (see **Table 28**)
2. Combination therapy with 2 or more agents with different actions
3. Add insulin hs or switch to insulin bid (see **Table 29**)
Manage hypertension (BP goal < 130/80 mm Hg; also see p 25) and lipid disorders (p 24; treat as CHD risk equivalent), as appropriate. ACE inhibitor or angiotensin II receptor blocker if albuminuria or proteinuria. Daily aspirin 81–325 mg.

Table 28. Oral Agents for Treating Diabetes Mellitus			
Drug	**Dosage**	**Formulations**	**Comments (Metabolism)**
2nd-Generation Sulfonylureas			Stimulate insulin secretion
Glimepiride (*Amaryl*)	4–8 mg once, begin 1–2 mg	[T: 1, 2, 4]	Numerous drug interactions, long-acting (L, K)
Glipizide (generic or *Glucotrol*)	2.5–40 mg once or divided	[T: 5, 10]	Short-acting (L, K)
(*Glucotrol XL*)	5–20 mg once	[SR: 2.5, 5, 10]	Long-acting (L, K)
Glyburide (generic or *Diaβeta, Micronase*)	1.25–20 mg once or divided	[T: 1.25, 2.5, 5]	Long-acting, risk of hypoglycemia (L, K)
Micronized glyburide (*Glynase*)	1.5–12 mg once	[T: 1.5, 3, 4.5, 6]	(L, K)
α-Glucosidase Inhibitors			Delay glucose absorption
Acarbose (*Precose*)	50–100 mg tid, just before meals, start with 25 mg	[T: 25, 50, 100]	GI side effects common, avoid if creatinine > 2 mg/dL, monitor LFTs (gut, K)
Miglitol (*Glyset*)	25–100 mg tid, with 1st bite of meal; start with 25 mg qd	[T: 25, 50, 100]	Same as acarbose but no need to monitor LFTs (L, K)

Table 28. Oral Agents for Treating Diabetes Mellitus (cont.)

Drug	Dosage	Formulations	Comments (Metabolism)
Biguanides			Insulin sensitizers
Metformin (*Glucophage*) XR	500–2550 divided 1500–2000 qd	[T: 500, 850, 1000] [T: ER 500, SR 500]	Avoid in patients > 80 yr, Cr, > 1.5 in men, Cr > 1.4 in women, CHF, COPD, ↑ LFTs (K)
Meglitinide			Increase insulin secretion
Nateglinide (*Starlix*)	60–120 mg tid	[T: 60, 120]	Give 30 min before meals
Repaglinide (*Prandin*)	0.5 mg bid–qid if HbA$_{1c}$ < 8% or previously untreated 1–2 mg bid–qid if HbA$_{1c}$ ≥ 8% or previously treated	[T: 0.5, 1, 2]	Give 30 min before meals, adjust dose at wkly intervals; potential for drug interactions, caution in liver, renal insufficiency (L)
Thiazolidinediones			Insulin resistance reducers; avoid if NYHA Class III or IV cardiac status; D/C if any decline in cardiac status
Pioglitazone (*Actos*)	15 or 30 mg qd; max 45 mg/d as monotherapy, 30 mg/d in combination therapy	[T: 15, 30, 45]	Check LFTs at start, q 2 mo during 1st yr, then periodically; avoid if clinical evidence of liver disease or if serum ALT levels > 2.5 upper limit of normal (L, K)
Rosiglitazone (*Avandia*)	4 mg qd–bid	[T: 2, 4, 8]	Check LFTs at start, q 2 mo during 1st yr, then periodically; avoid if clinical evidence of liver disease or if serum ALT levels > 2.5 upper limit of normal (L, K)
Combinations Glyburide & metformin (*Glucovance*)	1.25/250 mg initially if previously untreated; 2.5/500 mg or 5/500 mg bid with meals; maximum 20/2000/d	[T: 1.25/250, 2.5/500, 5/500]	Starting dose should not exceed the total daily dose of either drug; see also individual drugs

Table 29. Insulin Preparations			
Preparations	**Onset**	**Peak**	**Duration**
Insulin lispro	5–30 min	1–2 h	2–4 h
Insulin (eg, *Humulin, Novolin*)*			
Regular	1/2–1 h	2–4 h	4–6 h
NPH	2–4 h	8–12 h	24 h
Insulin aspart	15 min	45–90 min	3–5 h
(*Novolog*)			
Long-acting (eg, *Ultralente*)	4–8 h	10–30 h	> 36 h
Insulin glargine (*Lantus*)**	1–2 h	–	24 h

*Also available as mixtures of NPH and regular in 70:30 and 50:50 proportions.
** To convert from NPH dosing, give same number of units at bedtime. For patients taking NPH bid, decrease the total daily units by 20%, give at bedtime, and titrate on basis of response.

Monitoring (ADA)
- Weight, BP, and foot examination each visit
- HbA$_{1c}$ once or twice/yr in patients with stable glycemic control; quarterly, if poor control
- Annual comprehensive dilated eye and visual examinations by an ophthalmologist or optometrist who is experienced in management of diabetic retinopathy
- Lipid profiles every 1–2 yr depending on whether values are in normal range
- Annual (unless microalbuminuria has previously been demonstrated) test for microalbuminuria by measuring albumin-to-creatinine ratio in a random spot collection, timed collection, or 24-h collection

FALLS

DEFINITION
An event that results in a person's inadvertently coming to rest on the ground or lower level with or without loss of consciousness or injury. Excludes falls from major intrinsic event (seizure, stroke, syncope) or overwhelming environmental hazard.

ETIOLOGY
Typically multifactorial. Composed of intrinsic (eg, poor balance, visual or cognitive impairment), extrinsic (eg, polypharmacy), and environmental (eg, poor lighting, no safety equipment, loose carpets) factors. Commonly a nonspecific sign for one of many acute illnesses in older persons.

EVALUATION
Exclude acute illness or underlying systemic or metabolic process (eg, infection, electrolyte imbalance as indicated by history, examination, and laboratory studies). See **Figure 3** for recommended assessment and management.

History
- Circumstances of fall (eg, trip or slip, environmental hazard, recent meal)
- Associated symptoms (eg, lightheadedness, vertigo, syncope, weakness, confusion, palpitations)
- Relevant comorbid conditions (eg, prior stroke, parkinsonism, cardiac disease, seizure disorder, depression, anxiety, anemia, sensory deficit, osteoporosis, cognitive impairment)
- Previous falls
- Medication review, including OTC medications and alcohol use; note drugs that have hypotensive or psychoactive effects (see **Table 30**)

Physical
Look for:
- Vital signs: postural pulse and BP changes, fever, hypothermia
- Head and neck: visual impairment (especially poor acuity, reduced contrast sensitivity, decreased visual fields, cataracts), motion-induced imbalance (Dix-Hallpike test), bruit, nystagmus
- Musculoskeletal: arthritic changes, motion or joint limitations (especially lower extremity joint function), postural instability, skeletal deformities, podiatric problems
- Neurologic: slower reflexes, altered proprioception, altered mental status, focal deficits, peripheral neuropathy, gait or balance disorders, muscle weakness (especially leg), instability, tremor, rigidity
- Cardiovascular: heart arrhythmias, cardiac valve dysfunction
- Other: fever; hypothermia

Figure 3. Assessment and Management of Falls

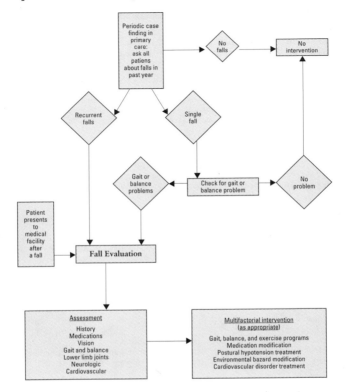

Source: American Geriatrics Society, British Geriatrics Society, and American Academy of Orthopaedic Surgeons Panel on Falls Prevention. Guideline for the prevention of falls in older persons. *J Amer Geriatr Soc.* 2001; 49(5):666. Reprinted with permission.

Functional Assessment

- Functional gait and balance: observe patient rising from chair, walking (stride length, velocity, symmetry), turning, sitting down (see also p 167)
- Mobility: observe the patient's use of assistive device (cane, walker, or personal assistance), extent of ambulation, restraint use

Ask about person's ability to complete activities of daily living: bathing, dressing, transferring, continence.

Table 30. Medications Associated With Increased Fall Risk		
Antiarrhythmics	Digoxin	Phenothiazines
Antihistamines	Diuretics	Sedative-hypnotics
Antihypertensives	Laxatives	Skeletal muscle relaxants
Antipsychotics	MAOIs	TCAs, SSRIs
Benzodiazepines	Opioids	Vasodilators

PREVENTION

Goal is to minimize risk of falling without compromising mobility and functional independence.

- Fall risk assessment should be part of every routine primary health care visit (at least annually).
- Assess for risk factors using a multidisciplinary approach, if appropriate, including medical and occupational therapy.
- Target interventions to risk factors (see **Table 31**). Correction of postural hypotension, review and modification of medications, and interventions to improve balance, transfers, and gait are priority.
- Choose fall prevention programs that include more than one intervention. A structured, interdisciplinary approach should be used.
  - Establish tailored exercise programs targeted at older people with mild deficits in strength, balance, lower extremity strength, and range of motion.
  - Tai Chi classes should be offered to older people living in the community.
  - Offer hip protectors to all residents of nursing homes—available via http://www.hipprotector.com, http://www.hipsaver.com, or http://safehip.com

Table 31. Risk Factors for Falls and Corresponding Interventions	
Risk Factor	**Interventions**
Postural hypotension: drop in SBP $\geq$ 20 mm Hg or to < 90 mm Hg on standing	Behavioral recommendations, such as ankle pumps or hand clenching and elevation of head of bed Decrease in dosage, discontinuation, or substitution of medication that may contribute to hypotension Pressure stockings (eg, Jobst) Fludrocortisone (*Florinef*) 0.1 mg qd–tid [0.1] if indicated Midodrine (*ProAmatine*) 2.5–5 mg tid [2.5, 5] Caffeinated coffee (1 cup) or caffeine 100 mg with meals
Use of any benzodiazepine or other sedative-hypnotic agent	Education about the appropriate use of sedative-hypnotic agents Nonpharmacologic treatment of sleep problems, eg, sleep restriction (see p 146) Tapering and discontinuation of medications

(continues)

Table 31. Risk Factors for Falls and Corresponding Interventions (cont.)	
Risk Factor	**Interventions**
Use of ≥ 4 prescription medications	Review and modification of medications, if appropriate
Environmental hazards for falls or tripping	Environment assessment with appropriate changes, eg: —removal of hazards —safer furniture (correct height, more stable) —installation of structures, eg, grab bars, handrails —improved lighting —reduced use of active restraints, eg, wheelchair adaptations, removable belts, wedge seating —protective hip padding
Any impairment in gait	Gait training Use of an appropriate assistive device Balance or strengthening exercises, if indicated
Any impairment in balance or transfer skills	Balance exercises; training in transfer skills, if indicated Environmental alterations, eg, grab bars, raised toilet seats
Impairment in leg or arm muscle strength or range of motion (hip, ankle, knee, shoulder, hand, elbow)	Exercises with resistive rubber bands and putty Resistance training 2–3 x/wk, increase resistance when able to complete 10 repetitions through the full range of motion Tai Chi

Source: Adapted from Tinetti ME, et al. A multifactorial intervention to reduce the risk of falling among elderly people living in the community. *N Engl J Med.* 1994;331:821–827. Copyright © 1994 Massachusetts Medical Society. All rights reserved. Adapted with permission.

GASTROESOPHAGEAL REFLUX DISEASE (GERD)
Definition
The retrograde movement of the gastric contents in the esophagus due to incompetent lower esophageal sphincter, transient relaxations of the sphincter, or compromise of other antireflux mechanisms.

Evaluation and Assessment
Empiric treatment is appropriate when hx typical for uncomplicated GERD.
- Endoscopy (if symptoms persist despite initial management, atypical presentation, or longstanding symptoms)
- 24-h pH monitoring

Warning Symptoms Suggesting Complicated GERD and Need For Diagnostic Evaluation
- Dysphagia
- Bleeding
- Weight loss
- Choking (acid causing cough, SOB, or hoarseness)
- Chest pain

Management
Nonpharmacologic:
- Antacids
- Avoid alcohol and fatty foods
- Avoid lying down 3 h after eating
- Avoid tight-fitting clothes
- Change diet (avoid pepper, spearmint, chocolate, spicy or acidic foods)
- Drink 6–8 oz water with all medications
- Elevate head of the bed (6–8 in)
- Lose weight (if overweight)
- Stop drugs that may promote reflux
- Stop smoking
- Surgery

Pharmacologic:

Table 32. Pharmacologic Management of GERD			
Drug	**Initial Oral Dosage**	**Maximum Dosage**	**Formulations (Excretion)**
Proton-Pump Inhibitors			
Esomeprazole (*Nexium*)	20 mg qd × 4 wk	–	[C: delayed release 20, 40] (L)
Lansoprazole (*Prevacid*)	15 mg qd × 8 wk	60 mg/d	[C: delayed-release 15, 30] (L)
Omeprazole (*Prilosec*)	20 mg qd × 4–8 wk	40 mg/d	[C: delayed-release 10, 20] (L)
Pantoprazole (*Protonix*)	40 mg qd × 8 wk	–	[T: 40]
Rabeprazole (*Aciphex*)	20 mg qd × 8 wk; 20 mg qd maintenance, if needed	–	[T: enteric-coated, delayed-release 20] (L)

(continues)

Table 32. Pharmacologic Management of GERD (cont.)			
Drug	Initial Oral Dosage	Maximum Dosage	Formulations (Excretion)
H₂ Antagonists (for less severe GERD)			
Cimetidine (*Tagamet*)	400 or 800 mg bid	1.5–2 × initial dose	[Inj; S: 200 mg/20 mL, 300 mg/ 5 mL with alcohol 2.8%; T: 100, 200,* 300, 400, 800] (K, L)
Famotidine (*Pepcid*)	20 mg bid × 6 wk	1.5–2 × initial dose	[Inj; oral susp. 40 mg/5 mL; T: film-coated 10,* 20, 40; C (gel): 10*; CT: 10*] (K)
Nizatidine (*Axid*)	150 mg bid	1.5–2 × initial dose	[C: 150, 300; T: 75] (K)
Ranitidine (*Zantac*)	150 mg bid	1.5–2 × initial dose	[C: (GELdose) 150, 300; granules, effervescent (EFFERdose) 150 mg; Inj; syrup 15 mg/mL; T: 75,* 150, 300; T: effervescent (EFFERdose) 150] (K, F)
Mucosal Protective Agent			
Sucralfate (*Carafate*)	1 g qid, 1h ac and hs	4 g/d	[Oral susp 1 g/10 mL; T: 1 g] (F, K)
Prokinetic Agents			
Bethanechol (*Urecholine*)	25 mg qid	50 mg qid	[Inj: 5 mg/mL; T: 5, 10, 25, 50] (unknown)
Metoclopramide† (*Reglan*)	5 mg qid, ac, and hs	15 mg qid	[Inj: 5 mg/mL; syrup, sugar-free: 5 mg/5 mL; T: 5, 10] (K, F)

* OTC strength.
† Risk of extrapyramidal symptoms high in persons aged > 65 yr.
Source: Data from DeVault KR, Castell DO. Updated guidelines for the diagnosis and treatment of gastroesophageal reflux disease. *Am J Gastroenterol.* 1999;94:1430–1442.

PEPTIC ULCER DISEASE
Causes
Helicobacter pylori is the major cause of peptic ulcer disease. NSAIDs are the second most common cause.

Diagnosis of *H pylori*
• Endoscopic examination   • Serology   • Urea breath test

Initial Treatment Options
• Empiric anti-ulcer treatment for 6 wk
• Definitive diagnostic evaluation by endoscopy
• Noninvasive testing for *H pylori* and treatment with antibiotics for (+) patients (see **Table 33** for regimens)
• Review patient's chronic medications for drug interactions before selecting regimen; many potential drug interactions and adverse drug reactions.

Table 33. FDA-Approved Treatments for *H pylori*–Induced Ulcerations (all oral routes)

Table 33. FDA-Approved Treatments for *H pylori*–Induced Ulcerations (all oral routes)
Lansoprazole 30 mg bid + amoxicillin 1 g bid + clarithromycin 500 mg tid × 10 (or 14) d
OR
Omeprazole 20 mg bid + clarithromycin 500 mg bid + amoxicillin 1 g bid × 10 d
OR
Lansoprazole 30 mg bid + clarithromycin 500 mg bid + amoxicillin 1 g bid × 10 d (*Prevpac*)
OR
Omeprazole 40 mg qd + clarithromycin 500 mg tid × 2 wk, then omeprazole 20 mg qd × 2 wk
OR
Lansoprazole 30 mg tid + amoxicillin 1 g bid × 2 wk (only for person allergic or intolerant to clarithromycin)
OR
Ranitidine bismuth citrate (RBC) 400 mg bid + clarithromycin 500 mg tid × 2 wk, then RBC 400 mg bid × 2 wk
OR
RBC 400 mg bid + clarithromycin 500 mg bid × 2 wk, then RBC 400 mg bid × 2 wk
OR
Bismuth subsalicylate (*Pepto-Bismol*) 525 mg qid (pc and hs) + metronidazole 250 mg qid + tetracycline 500 mg qid × 2 wk (*Helidac*) + H₂ receptor antagonist therapy as directed × 4 wk

Source: www.cdc.gov/ulcer/md.htm.
For additional, non-FDA approved regimens, see Howden CW, Hunt RH. Guidelines for the management of *Helicobacter pylori* infection. *Am J Gastroenterol* 1998;93:2330–2338. or www.acg.gi.org.

Medications
Bismuth subsalicylate (*Pepto-Bismol*) [CT: 262; suspension 262 mg/15 mL]
Antibiotics: (for complete information, see **Table 48**)
Amoxicillin (*Amoxil*) [C: 250, 500; CT: 125, 250; suspension 125 mg/5 mL, 250 mg/5 mL]
Clarithromycin (*Biaxin*) [T: film-coated 250, 500; oral suspension 125 mg/5 mL, 250 mg/5 mL]
Metronidazole (*Flagyl*) [T: 250, 500, 750; C: 375]
Tetracycline (*Achromycin, Sumycin*) [T: 250, 500; suspension 125 mg/5 mL]
Proton-Pump Inhibitors: See **Table 32**.
H₂ Antagonist Combination:
Ranitidine bismuth citrate [ranitidine 162 mg, trivalent bismuth 128 mg, and citrate 110 mg] (*Tritec*) [T: 400]

CONSTIPATION
Definition
Infrequent, incomplete, or painful evacuation of feces.

Drugs That Constipate
- Analgesics—opiates
- Antacids with aluminum or calcium
- Anticholinergic drugs
- Antidepressants, lithium
- Antihypertensives
- Antipsychotics
- Barium sulfate
- Bismuth
- Calcium channel blockers
- Diuretics
- Iron

Conditions That Constipate

- Colon tumor or mechanical obstruction
- Dehydration
- Depression
- Diabetes mellitus
- Hypercalcemia
- Hypokalemia
- Hypothyroidism
- Immobility
- Low intake of fiber
- Panhypopituitarism
- Parkinson's disease
- Spinal cord injury
- Stroke
- Uremia

Table 34. Medications That May Relieve Constipation			
Medication	Onset of Action	Starting Dosage	Site and Mechanism of Action
Bisacodyl tab (*Dulcolax*)	0.25–1 h	5–15 mg × 1	Colon
Bisacodyl suppository (*Dulcolax*)		10 mg × 1	Colon
Docusate saline (*Colace*)	24–72 h	100 mg qd–qid	Small and large intestine; detergent activity; facilitates admixture of fat and water to soften stool
Lactulose (*Cephulac*)*		15–30 mL qd–bid	Colon: osmotic effect
Magnesium citrate (*Citroma*)	0.5–3 h	120–240 mL × 1	Small and large intestine; attracts, retains water in intestinal lumen
Magnesium hydroxide (*Milk of Magnesia*)		30 mL qd–bid	Osmotic effect and increased peristalsis in colon
Malt soup extract (*Maltsupex*)			Surfactant, stool softener; also reduces fecal pH
Methylcellulose psyllium (*Metamucil*)	12–24 h (up to 72 h)	1–2 rounded tsp or packets qd–tid with water or juice	Small and large intestine; holds water in stool; mechanical distention
Sodium phosphate/biphosphate emollient enema (*Fleet*)	2–15 min	1 4.5-oz enema × 1, repeat prn	Colon
Senna (*Senokot*)	6–10 h	2 tabs or 1 tsp qhs	Colon; direct action on intestine; stimulates myenteric plexus; alters water and electrolyte secretion
Sorbitol 70%	24–48 h	15–30 mL qd–bid	Colon; delivers osmotically active molecules to colon

* By prescription only.

NAUSEA AND VOMITING
Causes
- CNS disorders (eg, motion sickness, intracranial lesions)
- Drugs (eg, chemotherapy, NSAIDs, narcotic analgesics, antibiotics, digoxin)
- GI disorders (eg, mechanical obstruction; inflammation of stomach, intestine, or gallbladder; pseudoobstruction, motility disorders, dyspepsia, diabetic gastroparesis)
- Infections (eg, viral or bacterial gastroenteritis, hepatitis, otitis, meningitis)
- Metabolic conditions (eg, uremia, acidosis, hyperparathyroidism, adrenal insufficiency)
- Psychiatric disorders

Evaluation
- If patient is not seriously ill or dehydrated, can probably wait 24–48 h to see if symptoms resolve spontaneously.
- If patient is seriously ill, dehydrated, or has other signs of acute illness, hospitalize for further evaluation.
- If symptoms persist, evaluate according to suspected causes.

Pharmacologic Management
Drugs that are useful in the management of nausea and vomiting are listed in **Table 35**.

Table 35. Selected Antiemetics		
Drug	**Formulations**	**Dosages (Metabolism)**
Chlorpromazine (*Thorazine*)	[Concentrate: oral 30, 100 mg/mL; Inj; Sp: 25, 100 mg; syrup: 10 mg/5 mL; T: 10, 25]	Oral 10–25 mg q 4–6 h; IM, IV, 25–50 mg q 4–6 h; rectal 50–100 mg q 6–8 h (L)
Dimenhydrinate* (*Dramamine*)	[C: 50; Inj; S: 12.5 mg/4 mL, 16.62 mg/5 mL; T: 50; CT: 50]	Oral, IM IV: 50–100 mg q 4–6 h, not to exceed 400 mg/d (L)
Meclizine* (*Antivert*)	[C: 15, 25, 30; T: 12.5, 25, 50; CT: 25; T: film coated 25]	Motion sickness: 12.5–25 mg 1 h before travel, repeat dose q 12–24 h if needed; doses up to 50 mg may be needed; vertigo: 25–100 mg/d in divided doses (L)
Metoclopramide (*Reglan*)	[Inj; oral concentrate10 mg/mL; syrup, sugar-free, 5 mg/5 mL; T: 5, 10]	Chemotherapy-induced emesis, IV: 1–2 mg/kg 30 min before chemotherapy and q 2–4 to q 4–6 h; postoperative nausea and vomiting: IM 5–10 mg near the end of surgery (K)
Prochlorperazine (*Compazine*)	[C: sustained action: 10, 15, 30; Inj; Sp: 2.5, 5, 25; syrup 5 mg/5 mL; T: 5, 10, 25]	Oral or IM: 5–10 mg 3–4 times/d, usual maximum, 40 mg/d; IV: 2.5–10 mg; maximum 10 mg/dose or 40 mg/d; may repeat dose q 3–4 h as needed; rectal: 25 mg twice daily (L)

* Available OTC.
Note: All have potential CNS toxicity.

DIARRHEA
Causes
- Drugs (eg, antibiotics [see **Table 48**], laxatives, colchicine)
- Fecal impaction
- GI disorders (eg, irritable bowel syndrome, malabsorption, inflammatory bowel disease)
- Infections (eg, viral, bacterial, parasitic)
- Lactose intolerance

Evaluation
- If patient is not seriously ill or dehydrated and there is no blood in the stool, can probably wait 48 h to see if symptoms resolve spontaneously.
- If patient is seriously ill, dehydrated, or has other signs of acute illness, hospitalize for further evaluation.
- If diarrhea persists, evaluate on the basis of the most likely causes.

Pharmacologic Management
Drugs that are useful in the management of diarrhea are listed in **Table 36**.

Table 36. Antidiarrheals		
Drug	**Formulations**	**Dosage (Metabolism)**
Attapulgite* (*Kaopectate*)	[S: oral concentrate: 600, 750 mg/15 mL; T: 750; CT: 300, 600]	1200–1500 mg after each loose bowel movement or q 2 h; 15–30 mL up to 9 ×/d, up to 9000 mg/24 h (not absorbed)
Bismuth subsalicylate* (*Pepto-Bismol*)		2 tablets or 30 mL q 30 min to 1 h as needed up to 8 doses/24 h
Diphenoxylate with atropine (*Lomotil*)†	[S: oral: diphenoxylate hydrochloride 2.5 mg + atropine sulfate 0.025 mg/5 mL; T: diphenoxylate hydrochloride 2.5 mg and atropine sulfate 0.025 mg]	15–20 mg/d of diphenoxylate in 3–4 divided doses; maintenance 5–15 mg/d in 2–3 divided doses (L)
Loperamide* (*Imodium A-D*)	[Caplet, 2; C: 2; T: 2; S: oral: 1 mg/5 mL]	Initial: 4 mg (2 capsules), followed by 2 mg after each loose stool, up to 16 mg/d (8 capsules) (L)

* Available OTC.
† Potentially CNS toxic.

HEARING IMPAIRMENT

DEFINITION
The most common sensory impairment in old age. To quantify hearing ability, the necessary intensity (decibel = dB) and frequency (Hertz) of the perceived pure-tone signal must be described.

CLASSIFICATION
Table 38 gives the hearing levels associated with varying degrees of hearing loss.

Sensorineural Hearing Loss
Due to cochlear or retrocochlear pathology; both air and bone conduction thresholds are increased; causes: aging, eighth nerve damage from syphilis, viral meningitis, trauma, vascular events to eighth nerve or cortical tracts, acoustic neuroma, Ménière's disease.

Presbycusis (Old-Age Hearing Loss, a Subtype of Sensorineural Loss):
• Mainly high-frequency loss   • Recruitment (an increase in sensation of loudness)
• Impaired speech discrimination

Conductive Hearing Loss
Occurs when sound transmission to inner ear is impaired; bone conduction better than air conduction; causes include: external or middle ear disorders, including otosclerosis; rheumatoid arthritis; Paget's disease.

Central Auditory Processing Disorder
Loss of speech discrimination in excess of that from loss in hearing sensitivity; involves the CNS; occurs in dementia and infrequently with presbycusis.

EVALUATION
Screening
• Note problems during conversation
• Ask about hearing dysfunction
• Use a standardized questionnaire (see p 166)
• Test with handheld audioscope
• Use whisper test–stand behind patient 2 ft from ear, cover untested ear, fully exhale, whisper an easily answered question
• Refer patients who screen positive for audiologic evaluation

Audiometry
• Documents the dB loss across frequencies
• Determines the pattern of loss (see Classification, above)
• Determines if loss is unilateral or bilateral
  Note: If speech discrimination is less than 50%, results with hearing aids may be poor

Aggravating Factors
• Sensorineural loss—medication ototoxicity (eg, aminoglycosides, loop diuretics, cisplatin), cerumen impaction (see **Table 37**)
• Conductive loss—cerumen impaction, external otitis

Table 37. Ear Wax Removal

Agent	Dosage	Comments
Ceruminolytic drops		
Carbamide peroxide (*Debrox, Murine Ear Drops, Cerumenex*)	5–10 drops each ear bid, cover with cotton × 4 d; liquid must stay in contact with ear for at least 15 min	Hearing may worsen as ear wax expands; use for longer than 7 d may cause irritation
Docusate sodium liquid (*Colace*)	See above	See above
Other agents		
Water	See above	Found in one controlled trial to be as effective as any commercial preparation
Olive oil	See above	

MANAGEMENT

Table 38. Effects and Rehabilitation of Hearing Loss, by Level of Loss

Level of Loss	Difficulty Understanding	Need for Hearing Aid
0–24 dB	None	None
25–40 dB (mild)	Normal speech	In specific situations
41–55 dB (moderate)	Loud speech	Frequent
56–80 dB (severe)	Anything but amplified speech	For all communication
81 dB or more (profound)	Even amplified speech	Plus speech reading, aural rehabilitation, or sign language

Source: Data in part from *A Report on Hearing Aids: User Perspectives and Concerns.* Washington, DC: American Association of Retired Persons; 1993:2.

Hearing Devices
Hearing Aids: Appropriate for most hearing-impaired persons; enhance select frequencies; should be individualized for each ear. Amplification in both ears (binaural) achieves best speech understanding; unilateral aid may be appropriate if asymmetrical speech discrimination or if hearing aid care is challenging.
Implantable Hearing Devices: Are FDA approved for adults with moderate to severe sensorineural hearing loss. Expensive.
Assistive Listening Devices: Microphone placed close to sound source transmits to headphones or earpiece. Transmission is by wire or wireless (FM or infrared); these systems increase signal-to-noise ratio, which is useful for persons with central auditory processing disorder.
Telephone Device for the Deaf (TDD): Receiver is a keyboard that allows the hearing-impaired person to respond.

Tips for Communication with Hearing-Impaired Persons
- Stand 2–3 ft away
- Have the person's attention
- Have the person seated in front of a wall, which will help reflect sound
- Use lower-pitched voice
- Speak slowly and distinctly; don't shout
- Rephrase rather than repeat
- Pause at the end of phrases or ideas

ANEMIA

Evaluation

- Some decrease in hemoglobin with age is normal.
- Evaluate persons > 65 when Hb < 12 in men and when Hb < 11.5 in women.
- Evaluate if Hb falls > 1 g/dL in 1 yr.
- Check reticulocyte count for hypo- or hyperregenerative disorder (see **Table 39**).
- Obtain bone marrow aspirate and biopsy if causes not clear.

Treatment

Table 39. Diagnosis and Management of Anemia		
Anemia Type	**Findings & Considerations**	**Management**
Hyporegenerative		
Chronic disorders	Chronic underlying disease Normocytic or microcytic RBCs Absent sideroblasts in marrow Iron studies, heavy metal screen	Treat underlying disorder Erythropoietin 50–100 U/kg q wk; increase dose to 150 U/kg if no response in 2–3 wk
Iron deficiency	Absent bone marrow hemosiderin Serum ferritin ≤ 50 µg/L with transferrin saturation ≤ 0.08 Serum ferritin ≤ 20 µg/L	Correct cause of blood loss Oral iron supplements: ferrous sulfate 325 mg po qd; parenteral iron* if iron absorption poor or not tolerated
B_{12} deficiency	Macrocytosis, giant and multi- lobar neutrophils, ↓ platelets; serum B_{12}, folate, and TSH; methylmalonic and homocys- teine in selected patients**	B_{12} 1000 µg/wk × 5 wk, then 100 µg IM/ mo or 1000 µg po daily for life Potassium for the 1st wk and iron supplement if anemia is severe
Aplastic anemia	Pancytopenia; bone marrow aspirate and biopsy; tartrate- resistant acid phosphatase; bone marrow chromosomal analysis[†]	Consult hematology
Hyperregenerative		
Autoimmune hemolytic anemia	Microspherocytes, cold and warm agglutinating antibodies[‡]	Consult hematology
Microangiopathic hemolytic anemia	Circulating schistocytes, hemo- globinuria, hemosiderinuria[§]	Iron and folate replacement, and consult hematology

* Iron dextran: Dose (mL) = 0.0442 (desired Hb − observed Hb) × LBW (kg) + (0.26 × LBW). For LBW, see p 1.
Administer test dose at 0.5 cc IM or IV solution (5 gtt/min). If tolerated, complete dose by slow IM injection ≤ 50 mg/min.
By IV, dilute dose in 500 mL NS (45–60 cc/min).
**If level is borderline (200–300 pg/mL) and results would change treatment decision.
† For myelodysplastic anemias, clonal disorders with macrocytic red cells, and abnormal red cell precursors in bone marrow; five subtypes which determine outcome; primary treatment is supportive with blood component transfusions; erythropoietin may help; other therapy depends on subtype.
‡ Differential diagnosis: lymphocytic lymphoma, chronic lymphocytic leukemia, collagen vascular disease, infection, medication-induced idiopathic disease.
§ Differential diagnosis: diabetes mellitus, atherosclerosis, collagen vascular disease. Acute forms: hypertensive crisis, vasculitis, disseminated intravascular coagulation, thrombotic thrombocytopenic purpura.

CANCER

Many older persons receive long-term drug therapy for cancers of the breast and prostate.

Breast Cancer

Prevention: Also see **Table 66**. Tamoxifen 20 mg po qd reduces breast cancer risk by 49% in women at high risk. For risk assessment see http://cancernet.nci.nih.gov/brca_tool.html

Monitoring:
- History, physical
- LFTs, calcium every 4–6 mo for 5 yr, then yearly
- Annual mammography, pelvic, and FOBT

Pharmacotherapy: Postmenopausal women with estrogen receptor (ER) or progesterone receptor (PR) positive tumors at high risk for recurrence (tumors greater than 1 cm, or positive nodes) should be treated with tamoxifen or letrozole for 5 yr, even when treated with chemotherapy. See **Table 40**.

Adjuvant Chemotherapy: Reduces recurrence risk for receptor-negative tumors. There is an additional 5% to 10% reduction in recurrence in ER- or PR-positive tumors treated with both tamoxifen and chemotherapy.

Table 40. Oral Agents for Breast Cancer Treatment				
Agent	**Dosage**	**Formulations**	**Monitoring**	**Comment**
Tamoxifen* (*Nolvadex*)	20 mg po qd	[T: 10, 20]	Annual eye exam; endometrial cancer screening	Drug interactions: erythromycin, calcium channel blockers; ↑ risk of thrombosis
Letrozole*† (*Femara*)	2.5 mg po qd	[T: 2.5]	Periodic CBC, LFTs, TSH	First-line therapy for hormone-responsive metastatic disease or tamoxifen failure
Anastrazole† (*Arimidex*)	1 mg po qd	[T: 1]	Periodic CBC, LFTs, lipids	First-line therapy for hormone-responsive metastatic disease or tamoxifen failure; may have more side effects

* Reduce dose if CrCl < 10 mL/min.
† In head-to-head trials these aromatase inhibitors have lower recurrence rates than tamoxifen; both are more effective than tamoxifen in advanced inoperable disease.

Prostate Cancer

PSA: See **Table 66**.

Histology:
- Gleason score 2–6 has low 15–20 yr morbidity and mortality; watchful waiting usually appropriate.

- Gleason score ≥ 7, higher PSA and younger age associated with higher morbidity and mortality; best treatment strategy (surgery, radiation, androgen suppression, etc.) is not known.

Pharmacotherapy: Hormonal therapy is indicated in locally advanced $\geq$ stage III or T3 (tumor extension beyond the prostate capsule) and metastatic prostate cancer. Treatment of earlier stage disease is controversial. Drugs of choice are leuprolide or goserelin with or without flutamide.

Table 41. Common Drugs for Prostate Cancer Therapy			
Class, Agent	**Dosage**	**Metabolism**	**Side Effects**
LH-RH agonists			
Goserelin acetate implant (*Zoladex*)	3.6 mg SC q 28 d or 10.8 mg q 3 mo	Rapid urinary and hepatic excretion, no dose adjustment in renal impairment	Side effects: hot flushes (60%), breast swelling, libido change, impotence, nausea
Leuprolide acetate (*Lupron Depot*)	7.5 mg IM q mo or 22.5 mg q 3 mo or 30 mg q 4 mo	Unknown; active metabolites for 4–12 wk, dose-dependent	Certain symptoms (obstruction, spinal cord compression, bone pain) may be exacerbated early in treatment; side effects: hot flushes (60%), edema (12%), pain (7%), nausea, vomiting, impotence, dyspnea, asthenia (all 5%), thrombosis, PE, MI (all 1%); headache as high as 32%
Antiandrogens			
Bicalutamide (*Casodex*) [T: 50]	50 mg po qd	Metabolized in liver, excreted in urine; half-life 10 d at steady state	Class side effects: nausea, hot flushes, breast pain, gynecomastia, hematuria, diarrhea, liver enzyme elevations, galactorrhea; delayed light adaptation (nilutamide)
Flutamide (*Eulexin*)[C: 125]	125 mg cap 2 po q 8 h	Renally excreted; half-life 5–6 h	
Nilutamide (*Nilandron*) [T: 50]	300 mg for 30 d, then 150 mg po qd	80% protein bound; liver metabolism, renal excretion; half-life 40–60 h	

INFECTIOUS DISEASES

PNEUMONIA
Presentation
Can range from subtle signs such as lethargy, anorexia, dizziness, falls, and delirium to septic shock or adult respiratory distress syndrome. Pleuritic chest pain, dyspnea, productive cough, chills, or rigors are not consistently present in older patients.

Evaluation and Assessment
- Physical examination: Respiratory rate > 20 breaths/min; low BP, chest sounds may be minimal, absent, or be consistent with CHF; temperature: 20% will be afebrile.
- CXR: Infiltrate may not be present on initial film if the patient is dehydrated.
- Sputum Gram's stain and culture (optional per ATS guidelines)
- CBC with differential: Up to 50% of patients have a normal WBC, but 95% have a left shift.
- BUN, creatinine, electrolytes
- Blood culture $\times$ 2
- Oxygenation: arterial blood gas or oximetry
- Test for *Mycobacterium tuberculosis* with acid fast bacili strain and culture in selected patients.
- Test for *Legionella* spp in selected patients (seriously ill without an alternative diagnosis, immunocompromised, nonresponsive to β-lactam antibiotics, with clinical features suggesting this diagnosis, or in outbreak setting). Urinary antigen testing is highly specific for serotype 1 but lacks specificity for other serotypes. Value and use vary by geographic region.

Aggravating Factors
- Age-related changes in pulmonary reserve
- Alcoholism
- Altered mental status
- Comorbid conditions that alter gag reflexes or ciliary transport
- COPD or other lung disease
- Heart disease
- Malnutrition
- Medications: Immunosuppressants, sedatives, anticholinergic or other agents that dry secretions, agents that decrease gastric pH
- Nasogastric tubes

Expected Organisms (in order of frequency of occurrence)

Community-Acquired:	*Nursing-Home–Acquired:*	*Hospital-Acquired:*
Streptococcus pneumoniae	*S pneumoniae*	Gram-negative bacteria
Respiratory viruses	Gram-negative bacteria	Anaerobes
Haemophilus influenzae	*Staphylococcus aureus*	Gram-positive bacteria
Gram-negative bacteria	Anaerobes	Fungi
Moraxella catarrhalis	*H influenzae*	
Legionella spp	Group B streptococcus	
M tuberculosis	*Chlamydia pneumoniae*	
Endemic fungi		

70

Supportive Management
- Chest percussion
- Inhaled β-adrenergic agonists
- Mechanical ventilation (if indicated)
- Oxygen as indicated
- Rehydration

Empiric Antibiotic Therapy (see Table 48)

Community-Acquired (All Via Oral Route): [Second-generation cephalosporin or β-lactam/β-lactamase inhibitor or fluoroquinolone with enhanced activity against *S pneumoniae**] ± macrolide if *Legionella* spp suspected

Community-Acquired with Hospitalization (Oral or IV Route): [Second-, third-, or fourth-generation cephalosporin or β-lactam/β-lactamase inhibitor or fluoroquinolone with enhanced activity against *S pneumoniae**] ± erythromycin or other macrolide if *Legionella* spp suspected

Severe Community-Acquired with Hospitalization (IV Route Initially): Macrolide + ceftazidime or cefepime or another antipseudomonal agent

Nursing-Home–Acquired (IV Route): [(First- or second-generation cephalosporin or ureidopenicillin) + aminoglycoside] ± penicillin G, clindamycin, or vancomycin; *or* Third- or fourth-generation cephalosporin ± aminoglycoside ± penicillin G, clindamycin, or vancomycin; *or*
Ureidopenicillin + aminoglycoside; *or*
Vancomycin + clindamycin + aminoglycoside; *or*
For the oral route: See community-acquired pneumonia (all via oral route) ± quinolone.

Hospital-Acquired (IV Route): [Third- or fourth-generation cephalosporin + clindamycin or penicillin G] ± aminoglycoside; *or*
Ureidopenicillin + aminoglycoside or other antipseudomonal agent; *or*
First- or second-generation cephalosporin + aminoglycoside; *or*
Vancomycin + clindamycin + aminoglycoside; *or*
Ureidopenicillin + second-generation cephalosporin; *or*
β-lactam/β-lactamase inhibitor + antipseudomonal agent.
For hospital- or nursing-home–acquired pneumonia, a macrolide, tetracycline, or quinolone may be added or substituted when *Legionella* spp, *Chlamydia pneumoniae*, or *Mycoplasma pneumoniae* is suspected.

* Refers to levofloxacin, sparfloxacin, moxifloxacin.
Note: The empiric use of vancomycin should be reserved for patients with a serious allergy to β-lactam antibiotics or for patients from environments in which methicillin-resistant *S aureus* is known to be a problem pathogen. For all cases, antimicrobial therapy should be individualized once Gram's stain or culture results are known.

URINARY TRACT INFECTION OR UROSEPSIS
Definition
Bacteriuria: Presence of significant number of bacteria without reference to symptoms
UTI: Symptomatic bacteriuria

Table 42. Quantitative Urine Microbiology for Diagnosis of Urinary Tract Infection

Clinical Presentation	Quantitative Microbiology
Asymptomatic	Same organism(s) $\geq 10^5$ cfu/mL on 2 consecutive cultures
Pyelonephritis or fever with localized symptoms	$\geq 10^4$ cfu/mL
Acute lower tract symptoms	$\geq 10^3$ cfu/mL of uropathogen
Specimen collected from: External collecting device (men only) Aspirated indwelling catheter	$\geq 10^5$ cfu/mL $\geq 10^3$ cfu/mL

Source: Nicolle LE. Urinary tract infections in the elderly. In: Hazzard WR, Blass JP, Ettinger WH, et al., eds., *Principles of Geriatric Medicine and Gerontology*, 3rd ed. New York: McGraw-Hill Publishing; 1994. Reprinted with permission of The McGraw-Hill Companies.

Risk Factors
- Abnormalities in function or anatomy of the urinary tract
- Catheterization or recent instrumentation
- Comorbid conditions (eg, diabetes mellitus, BPH)
- Female gender
- Limited functional status

Assessment and Evaluation
Choice is based on presenting symptoms and severity of illness.
- Urinalysis with Gram's stain and culture
- Blood culture $\times$ 2
- BUN, creatinine, electrolytes
- CBC with differential

Expected Organisms
Noncatheterized Patients: Most common: *Escherichia coli, Proteus* spp, *Klebsiella* spp, *Providencia* spp, *Citrobacter* spp, *Enterobacter* spp, and *Pseudomonas aeruginosa* if recent antibiotic exposure, known colonization, or known institutional flora
Nursing-Home–Catheterized Patients: *Enterobacter* spp and gram-negative bacteria

Empiric Antibiotic Management
Duration should be at least 7–10 d.
Community-Acquired or Nursing-Home–Acquired Cystitis or Uncomplicated UTI (Oral Route): TMP/SMZ DS, cephalexin, ampicillin, or amoxicillin. Amoxicillin/clavulanic acid should be reserved for patients with sulfa allergy and in settings where β-lactam resistance is known. Fluoroquinolones should be reserved for patients with allergies to sulpha, β-lactams, or in settings where resistance is known.
Suspected Urosepsis (IV Route): Third-generation cephalosporin plus aminoglycoside, aztreonam, or fluoroquinolone $\pm$ aminoglycoside.

Vancomycin should be used in patients with severe β-lactam allergy and gram-positive chains or clusters in urine on Gram's stain.

HERPES ZOSTER ("SHINGLES")

Definition
Cutaneous vesicular eruptions followed by radicular pain secondary to the recrudescence of varicella zoster virus.

Clinical Manifestations
- An abrupt onset of pain along a specific dermatome (see **Figure 1**)
- Macular, erythematous rash after ~3 d which becomes vesicular and pustular (Tzanck cell test positive), crusts over and clears in 10–14 d
- Complications: post-herpetic neuralgia, visual loss or blindness if ophthalmic involvement

Pharmacologic Management
When started within 72 h of the rash's appearance, antiviral therapy decreases the severity and duration of the acute illness and possibly shortens the duration and reduces the risk of post-herpetic neuralgias. Corticosteroids may also decrease the risk and severity of post-herpetic neuralgias. (See p 103 for treatment of post-herpetic neuralgia.)

Table 43. Antiviral Treatments for Herpes Zoster			
Agent, Route	**Dosage**	**Formulations**	**Comment**
Acyclovir (*Zovirax*)			
Oral	800 mg 5 ×/d for 7–10 d	[T: 400, 800; C: 200; S: 200 mg/5 mL]	Adjust dose when CrCl* < 50 mL/min
IV**	10 mg/kg q 8 h for 7–10 d	[500 mg/10 mL]	
Famciclovir (*Famvir*)			
Oral	500 mg q 8 h for 7–10 d	[T: 125, 250, 500]	Adjust dose when CrCl* < 60 mL/min
Valacyclovir† (*Valtrex*)			
Oral	1000 mg q 8 h for 7–10 d	[C: 500, 1000]	Adjust dose when CrCl* < 50 mL/min

* The CrCl listed is the threshold below which the dose or frequency should be adjusted. See alternative reference or the drug's package insert for detailed dosing guidelines.
** Use IV for serious illness, ophthalmic infection, or patients who cannot take oral medication.
† Preferred to po acyclovir; pro-drug of acyclovir with serum concentrations equal to IV.

INFLUENZA

Vaccine Prevention (ACIP Guidelines)
Yearly vaccination is recommended for all persons ≥ 65 years and all residents and staff of nursing homes, or residential or long-term-care facilities. Nursing-home residents admitted during the winter months after the completion of the vaccination program should be vaccinated at admission if they have not already been vaccinated. The influenza vaccine is contraindicated in persons with an anaphylactic hypersensitivity to eggs or any other component of the vaccine. Dose: 0.5 mL IM × 1 in the fall (Oct–Nov) for residents in the northern hemisphere.

Pharmacologic Prophylaxis and Treatment with Antiviral Agents
Indications:
- Prevention (during an influenza outbreak): persons who are not vaccinated, are immunodeficient, or may spread the virus
- Prophylaxis: during 2 wk required to develop antibodies for persons vaccinated after an outbreak of influenza A
- Reduction of symptoms, duration of illness when started within the first 48 h of symptoms
- During epidemic outbreaks in nursing homes

Duration: Treatment of symptoms: 3–5 d or for 24–48 h after symptoms resolve. Prophylaxis during an outbreak: Minimum 2 wk or until ~1 wk after the end of the outbreak.

Table 44. Antiviral Treatment of Influenza

Agent	Dosage
Amantadine (*Symmetrel*)	100 mg po daily*
Oseltamivir (*Tamiflu*)**	Treatment: 75 mg po bid × 5 d (75 mg po qd if CrCl 10–30 mL/min) Prophylaxis: 75 mg po qd × ≥ 7 d up to 2 wk (75 mg po qod if CrCl 10–30 mL/min)
Rimantadine (*Flumadine*)	100 mg po qd for frail elderly and nursing-home residents 200 mg po qd for other adults, including those ≥ 65 yr Decrease dose to 100 mg if side effects appear
Zanamivir (*Relenza*)**†	2 × 5–mg inhalations q 12 h × 5 d Give doses on 1st d at least 2 h apart

*Dose adjustments for renal function, CrCl (mL/min): ≥ 30 = 100 mg daily; 20–29 = 200 mg 2 ×/wk; 10–19 = 100 mg 3 ×/wk; < 10 = 200 mg alternating with 100 mg q 7 d.
** Must be started within 2 d of symptom onset.
† Do not use in patients with COPD or asthma.

INFECTIOUS TUBERCULOSIS
Tuberculosis (TB) in elderly patients may be the reactivation of old disease or a new infection due to exposure to an infected individual. Treatment recommendations differ, and if a new infection is suspected or the patient has risk factors for resistant organisms, bacterial sensitivities must be determined (see **Table 46**).

Risk or Reactivating Factors
- Chronic institutionalization
- Corticosteroid use
- Diabetes mellitus
- Malignancy
- Malnutrition
- Renal failure

Risk Factors for Resistant Organisms
- HIV infection
- Homelessness, institutionalization (other than a nursing home)
- IV drug abuse
- Origin from geographic regions with a high prevalence of resistance (New York, Mexico, Southeast Asia)
- Exposure to INH-resistant TB or history of failed chemotherapy
- Previous treatment for TB
- AFB-positive sputum smears after 2 mo of treatment
- Positive cultures after 4 mo of treatment

Diagnosis
• PPD with booster 5-TU subdermal; read in 48–72 h; repeat in 1–2 wk if negative
• CXR

Treatment

Table 45. Identification of Patients at High Risk of Developing TB Who Would Benefit From Treatment of Latent Infection	
Population	**Minimum Induration Considered a Positive Test**
Low risk: testing generally not indicated	15 mm
Residents and employees of hospitals, nursing homes, and long-term facilities for elderly persons, residential facilities for AIDS patients, and homeless shelters Recent immigrants (< 5 yr) from high-prevalence countries Injection drug users Persons with silicosis, diabetes mellitus, chronic renal failure, leukemia, lymphoma, carcinoma of the head, neck, or lung, weight loss of ≥ 10%, gastrectomy or jejunoileal bypass	10 mm
Recent contact with TB patients Fibrotic changes on CXR consistent with prior TB Immunosuppressed (receiving the equivalent of ≥ 15 mg/d of prednisone for ≥ 1 mo) or organ transplants HIV-positive patients	5 mm

Table 46. Treatment of Latent Tuberculosis	
Drug	**Dose and Duration**
Isoniazid*	5 mg/kg/d (maximum 300 mg/d) for 6 or 9 mo; or 15 mg/kg/d (maximum 900 mg/d) 2 ×/wk with directly observed therapy (DOT) for 6 or 9 mo
Rifampin plus Pyrazinamide†	10 mg/kg/d (maximum 600 mg/d) 15–20 mg/kg/d (maximum 2 gm/d) daily for 2 mo
or	
Rifampin plus Pyrazinamide†	10 mg/kg/d (maximum 600 mg/d) 2 ×/wk with DOT for 2–3 mo 50 mg/kg/d (maximum 4 gm/d) 2 ×/wk with DOT for 2–3 mo
Rifampin	10 mg/kg/d (maximum 600 mg/d) for 4 mo

* The preferred treatment for patients not infected with HIV.
† Use the combination therapy with caution, as the 2-mo regimen has been associated with liver injury. Obtain a serum aminotransferase, and bilirubin at baseline and 2, 4, and 6 wk of treatment. For additional information, see *MMWR* 2001; 50(34):733–735 or http://www.ajrccm.atsjournals.org/cgi/content/full/161/4/S1/S221/DC1
Source: Data from: American Thoracic Society. Targeted tuberculin testing and treatment of latent tuberculosis. *Am J Respir Crit Care Med* 2000;161:S221–S247 (also available at http://www.atsjournal.org).

ANTIBIOTIC-ASSOCIATED DIARRHEA
(Antibiotic-associated pseudomembranous colitis, or AAPMC)

Definition
A specific form of *Clostridium difficile* pseudomembranous colitis

Risk Factors
Almost any oral or parenteral antibiotic and several antineoplastic agents, including cyclophosphamide, doxorubicin, fluorouracil, methotrexate.

Presentation
• Abdominal pain, cramping
• Dehydration
• Diarrhea (can be bloody)
• Fecal leukocytes
• Fever (100–105°F)
• Hypoalbuminemia
• Hypovolemia
• Leukocytosis

Symptoms appear a few days after starting to 10 wk after discontinuing the offending agent.

Diagnosis
• Isolation of *C difficile* or its toxin from symptomatic patient.
• Lower endoscopy; however, lesions may be scattered.

Treatment
• Discontinue offending agent if possible.
• Metronidazole (*Flagyl*) 250 mg po qid or 500 mg po tid × 10 d or vancomycin 125–500 mg po qid × 10 d.
• Treat diarrhea with cholestyramine resin (eg, *Questran*) 4 g 1–6 ×/d to adsorb toxin.
• Avoid opiates or other agents that will slow GI motility.

Recurrence
Relapse seen in 10% to 20% of patients 1–4 wk after treatment (spore-producing organism). Re-treat with same regimen or use alternative.

Table 47. Monitoring Aminoglycosides and Vancomycin		
Antimicrobial	**Therapeutic Concentration**	
	Peak (µg/mL)	**Trough (µg/mL)**
Amikacin	25–30	4–8 (< 5*)
Gentamicin or tobramycin	4–8	< 2 (< 0.5*)
Vancomycin	20–40	5–10

* For once-daily or extended-interval dosing.

Table 48. Antibiotics				
Class, *Subclass*, Antimicrobial	Route of Elimination (%)	Dosage	Adjust When CrCl* Is: (mL/min)	Formulations
β–Lactams				
Penicillins				
Amoxicillin (*Amoxil*)	K (80)	po: 250 mg–1 g q 8 h	< 50	[T: film coated -500, 875] [C: 250, 500] [CT: 125, 200, 250, 400] [S: 125, 200, 250, 400 mg/5 mL]
Ampicillin	K (90)	po: 250–500 mg q 6 h IM/IV: 1–2 g q 4–6 h	< 30	[C: 250, 500] [S: 125, 250 mg/5 mL] [Inj]
Penicillin G	K L (30)	IV: 3–5 × 10⁶ U q 4–6 h IM: 0.6–2.4 × 10⁶ U q 6–12 h	< 30	[Inj] [Procaine for IM]
Penicillin VK	K, L	po: 125–500 mg q 6 h		[T: 125, 250, 500] [S: 125, 250 mg/5 mL]
Carbenicillin indanyl sodium (*Geocillin*)	K (80–99)	po: 382–764 mg q 6 h	< 50	[T: 382]
Ureidopenicillins				
Mezlocillin (*Mezlin*)	K	IM: 1–2 g q 8–12 h IV: 2 g q 6–8 h	< 30	[Inj]
Penicillinase-resistant Nafcillin (*Nafcil*)	L	po: 250 mg–1 g q 4–6 h IM: 500 mg q 4–6 h IV: 500 mg–2 g q 4–6 h	NA	[C: 250] [T: 500] [S: 250 mg/5 mL] [Inj]
Oxacillin (*Bactocill*)	K	po: 500 mg–1 g q 4–6 h IM, IV: 250 mg–2 g q 6–12 h	< 10	[C: 250, 500] [S: 250 mg/5 mL] [Inj]
Aztreonam (*Azactam*)	K (70)	IM: 500 mg–1 g q 8–12 h IV: 500 mg–2 g q 6–12 h	< 30	[Inj]
Meropenem (*Merrem IV*)	K (75) L (25)	IV: 1 g q 8 h	≤ 50	[Inj]
Imipenem-Cilastatin (*Primaxin*)	K (70)	IM: 500 mg–1 g q 8–12 h IV: 500 mg–2 g q 6–12 h	< 70	[Inj]
Amoxicillin–Clavulanate (*Augmentin*)	K	po: 250 mg q 8 h, 500 mg q 12 h, 875 mg q 12 h	< 30	[T: 250, 500, 875] [CT: 125, 200, 250, 400] [S: 125, 200, 250, 400 mg/5 mL]

(*continues*)

Table 48. Antibiotics (cont.)				
Class, *Subclass*, Antimicrobial	Route of Elimination (%)	Dosage	Adjust When CrCl* Is: (mL/min)	Formulations
Ampicillin–Sulbactam (*Unasyn*)	K (85)	IM, IV: 1–2 g q 6–8 h	< 30	[Inj]
Piperacillin–Tazo- bactam (*Zosyn*)	K	IV: 3.375 g q 6 h	< 40	[Inj]
Ticarcillin–Clavu- lanate (*Timentin*)	K, L	IV: 3 g q 4–6 h	< 60	[Inj]
First-Generation Cephalosporins				
Cefadroxil (*Duricef*)	K (90)	po: 500 mg–1 g q 12 h	< 50	[C: 500; T: 1 g] [S: 125, 250, 500 mg/ 5 mL]
Cefazolin (*Ancef, Kefzol*)	K (80–100)	IM, IV: 500 mg–2 g q 8 h	< 55	[Inj]
Cephalexin (*Keflex*)	K (80–100)	po: 250 mg–1 g q 6 h	< 40	[C: 250, 500] [T: 250, 500; 1 g] [S: 125, 250 mg/5 mL]
Cephalothin (*Keflin*)	K (50–75)	IM, IV: 500 mg–2 g q 4–6 h	< 50	[Inj]
Cephapirin (*Cefadyl*)	K (60–85)	IM, IV: 1–3 g q 6 h	< 10	[Inj]
Cephradine (*Anspor*)	K (80–90)	po, IM, IV: 500 mg– 2 g q 6 h	< 20	[C: 250, 500] [T: 1 g] [S: 125, 250 mg/5 mL] [Inj.]
Second-Generation Cephalosporins				
Cefaclor (*Ceclor*)	K (80)	po: 250–500 mg q 8 h	< 50	[C: 250, 500] [S: 125, 187, 250, 375 mg/ 5 mL] [T: ER–375, 500]
Cefamandole (*Mandol*)	K	IM, IV: 1–3 g q 6 h	< 80	[Inj]
Cefmetazole (*Zefazone*)	K (85)	IV: 2 g q 6–12 h	< 90	[Inj]
Cefotetan (*Cefotan*)	K (80)	IM, IV: 1–3 g q 12 h or 1–2 g q 24 h (UTI)	< 30	[Inj]
Cefoxitin (*Mefoxin*)	K (85)	IM, IV: 1–2 g q 6–8 h	< 50	[Inj]
Cefprozil (*Cefzil*)	K (60–70)	po: 250–500 mg q 12–24 h	< 30	[T: 250, 500] [S: 125, 250 mg/5 mL]

Table 48. Antibiotics (cont.)				
Class, *Subclass*, Antimicrobial	Route of Elimination (%)	Dosage	Adjust When CrCl* Is: (mL/min)	Formulations
Cefuroxime axetil (*Ceftin*)	K (66–100)	po: 125–500 mg q 12 h IM, IV: 750 mg–1.5 g q 6 h		[T: 125, 250, 500] [S: 125, 150 mg/5 mL] [Inj]
Loracarbef (*Lorabid*)	K	po: 200–400 mg q 12–24 h	< 50	[C: 200, 400] [S: 100, 200 mg/5 mL]
Third-Generation Cephalosporins				
Cefdinir (*Omnicef*)	K	po: 300 mg bid or 600 qd × 10 d	< 30	[C: 300] [S: 125 mg/5 mL]
Cefixime (*Suprax*)	K (50)	po: 400 mg q 24 h	< 60	[T: 200, 400] [S: 100 mg/5 mL]
Cefoperazone (*Cefobid*)	L, K (25)	IM, IV: 1–2 g q 12 h	Adjust in cirrhosis	[Inj]
Cefotaxime (*Claforan*)	K, L	IM, IV: 1–2 g q 6–12 h	< 20	[Inj]
Cefpodoxime (*Vantin*)	K (80)	po: 100–400 mg q 12 h	< 30	[T: 100, 250] [S: 50, 100 mg/5 mL]
Ceftazideme (*Ceptaz, Fortaz*)	K	IM, IV: 500 mg–2 g q 8–12 h UTI: 250–500 mg q 12 h	< 50	[Inj]
Ceftibuten (*Cedax*)	K (65–70)	po: 400 mg q 24 h	< 50	[C: 400] [S: 100, 200 mg/5 mL]
Ceftizoxime (*Cefizox*)	K (100)	IM, IV: 500 mg–2 g q 4–12 h	< 80	[Inj]
Ceftriaxone (*Rocephin*)	K (33–65)	IM, IV: 1–2 g q 12–24 h	NA	[Inj]
Fourth-Generation Cephalosporins				
Cefepime (*Maxipime*)	K (85)	IV: 500 mg–2 g q 12 h	< 60	[Inj]
Aminoglycosides (see **Table 47** for monitoring levels)				
Amikacin (*Amikin*)	K (95)	IM, IV: 15–20 mg/kg/d divided q 12–24 h; 15–20 mg/kg q 24–48 h		[Inj]
Gentamicin (*Garamycin*)	K (95)	IM, IV: 2–5 mg/kg/d divided q 12–24 h; 5–7 mg/kg q 24–48 h		[Inj] [Ophth susp, ointment]

(*continues*)

Table 48. Antibiotics (cont.)				
Class, *Subclass,* Antimicrobial	Route of Elimination (%)	Dosage	Adjust When CrCl* Is: (mL/min)	Formulations
Streptomycin	K (90)	IM, IV: 10 mg/kg/d not to exceed 750 mg/d	< 50	[Inj]
Tobramycin (*Nebcin*)	K (95)	IM, IV: 2–5 mg/kg/d divided q 12–24 h; 5–7 mg/kg q 24–48 h		[Inj] [Ophth susp, ointment]
Macrolides				
Azithromycin (*Zithromax*)	L	po: 500 mg day 1, then 250 mg IV: 500 mg qd	NA	[C: 250] [S: 100, 200/5 mL, 1 g (single-dose packet)] [T: 600]
Clarithromycin (*Biaxin, Biaxin XL*)	L K (20–30)	po: 250–500 mg q 12 h XL: 1000 mg q 24 h	< 30	[S: 125, 250 mg/5 mL] [T: 250, 500] [SR(XL): 500]
Dirithromycin (*Dynabac*)	L, F	po: 500 mg qd with food	NA	[T: 250]
Erythromycin	L	po: Base: 333 mg q 8 h Estolate, stearate or base: 250–500 mg q 6–12 h Ethylsuccinate: 400–800 mg q 6–12 h IV: 15–20 mg/kg/d divided q 6 h	NA	[Base: C, T: 250, 333, 500] [Estolate: 250] [S: 125, 250 mg/5 mL] [T: 500] Ethylsuccinate: [S: 100, 200, 400 mg/5 mL] [T: 400] [CT: 200] [Stearate: T: 250, 500] [Inj]
Quinolones				
Cinoxacin (*Cinobac*)	K (60)	po: 500 bid	< 80	[C: 250, 500]
Ciprofloxacin (*Cipro*)	K (30–50) L, F (20–40)	po: 250–750 mg q 12 h IV: 200–400 mg q 12 h Ophth: see Table 80	po: < 50 IV: < 30	[T: 100, 250, 500, 750] [S: 250 mg/5 mL, 500 mg/5 mL] [Ophth sol'n: 3.5 mg/ 5 mL] [Inj]
Enoxacin (*Penetrex*)	K L (15–20)	po: 200 mg q 12 h × 7d or 400 mg q 12 h × 14 d	≤ 30	[T: 200, 400]
Gatifloxacin (*Tequin*)	K (95) F (5)	po, IV: 200–400 mg qd × 7–10 d	< 40	[T: 200, 400] [Inj]

Table 48. Antibiotics (cont.)				
Class, *Subclass*, Antimicrobial	Route of Elimination (%)	Dosage	Adjust When CrCl* Is: (mL/min)	Formulations
Levofloxacin (*Levaquin*)	K	po, IV: 250–500 mg q 24 h	< 50	[T: 250, 500]
Lomefloxacin (*Maxaquin*)	K	po: 400 mg q 24 h	< 40	[T: 400]
Moxifloxacin (*Avelox*)	L (~55), F (25), K (20)	po: 400 mg q 24 h	NA	[T: 400]
Norfloxacin (*Noroxin*)	K (30) F (30)	po: 400 mg q 12 h Ophth: see Table 80	< 30	[T: 400] [Ophth: 0.3%]
Ofloxacin (*Roxin*)	K	po, IV: 200–400 mg q 12–24 h Ophth: see Table 80	< 50	[T: 200, 300, 400] [Ophth: 0.3%] [Inj]
Sparfloxacin (*Zagam*)	L	po: 400 mg day 1, then 200 mg q 24 h	< 50	[T: 200]
Trovafloxacin (*Trovan*)	L	po, IV: 200 mg q 24 h × 10–14 d	NA	[T: 100, 200] [Inj.]
Tetracyclines				
Doxycycline (*Vibramycin*)	K (25) F (30)	po, IV: 100–200 mg/d given q 12–24 h	NA	[C: 50, 100] [T: 50, 100] [S: 25 mg/5 mL, 50 mg/5 mL] [Inj]
Minocycline (*Minocin*)	K	po, IV: 200 mg × 1, 100 mg q 12 h	NA	[C: 50, 100] [S: 50 mg/5 mL] [Inj]
Tetracycline	K (60)	po, IV: 250–500 mg q 6–12 h	NA	[C: 100, 250, 500] [T: 250, 500] [S: 125 mg/5 mL] [Ophth: ointment, susp] [Topical: ointment, solution]
Other Antibiotics				
Chloramphenicol (*Chloromycetin*)	L (90)	po, IV: 50 mg/kg/d given q 6 h; maximum: 4 g/d		[C: 250] [Topical] [Ophth] [Inj]
Clindamycin (*Cleocin*)	L (90)	po: 150–450 mg q 6–8 h; maximum: 1.8 g/d IM, IV: 1.2–1.8 g/d given q 8–12 h; maximum: 3.6 g/d	NA	[C: 75, 150, 300] [S: 75 mg/5 mL] [Cream, vaginal: 2%] [Gel, topical: 1%] [Inj]

(*continues*)

Table 48. Antibiotics (cont.)				
Class, *Subclass*, Antimicrobial	Route of Elimination (%)	Dosage	Adjust When CrCl* Is: (mL/min)	Formulations
Cotrimoxazole (TMP/SMZ, *Bactrim*)	K, L	Doses based on the trimethoprim component: po: 1 double-strength tablet q 12 h. IV: sepsis: 20 TMP/kg/d given q 6 h	≤ 50	[T: SMZ 400; TMP 80] [Double-strength: SMZ 800; TMP 160] [S: SMZ 200; TMP 40 mg/5 mL] [Inj]
Linezolid (*Zyvox*)	L (65) K (30)	po: 400–600 mg q12 h IV: 600 mg q 12 h	NA	[T: 400, 600] [S: 100 mg/5 mL] [Inj]
Metronidazole (*Flagyl, MetroGel*)	L (30–60) K (20–40) F (6–15)	po: 250–750 mg q 6–8 h Vaginal: 1 applicator full (375 mg) qhs or bid Topical: Apply bid	≤ 10	[T: 250, 500] [ER: 750] [C: 375] [Gel, topical: 0.75% (30g)] [Gel, vaginal: 0.75% (70g)] [Inj]
Nitrofurantoin (*Macrodantin*)	L (60) K (40)	po: 50–100 mg q 6 h	Do not use if < 40	[C: 25, 50, 100] [S: 25 mg/5 mL]
Quinupristin/ dalfopristin (*Synercid*)	L, B, F (75) K (15–19)	Vancomycin-resistant *E faecium*: IV: 7.5 mg/ kg q 8 h Complicated skin or skin structure infection: 7.5 mg/kg q 12 h	NA	[Inj]
Vancomycin (*Vancocin*) (see **Table 47** for monitoring levels)	K (80–90)	po: *C difficile*: 125–500 mg q 6–8 h IV: 500 mg–1 g q 8–24 h		[C: 125, 250] [Inj]
Antifungals				
Amphotericin B (*Fungizone*)	K	IV: test dose: 1 mg infused over 20–30 min; if tolerated, initial therapeutic dose is 0.25 mg/kg; the daily dose can be increased by 0.25-mg/kg increments on each subsequent day until the desired daily dose is reached Maintenance dose: IV: 0.25–1 mg/kg/d or 1.5 mg/kg qod; do not exceed 1.5 mg/kg/d	**	[Topical: cream, lotion, ointment 3%] [Inj]
Fluconazole (*Diflucan*)	K (80)	po, IV: first dose 200– 400 mg, then 100– 400 mg qd for 14 d–12 wk, depending on indication. Vaginal candidiasis: 150 mg as a single dose	< 50	[T: 50, 100, 150, 200] [S: 10 and 40 mg/mL] [Inj]

Table 48. Antibiotics (cont.)				
Class, *Subclass*, Antimicrobial	Route of Elimination (%)	Dosage	Adjust When CrCl* Is: (mL/min)	Formulations
Flucytosine (*Ancobon*)	K (75–90)	po: 50–150 mg/kg/d divided q 6 h	< 50	[C: 250, 500]
Griseofulvin (*Fulvicin P/G, Grifulvin V*)	L	po: Microsize: 500–1000 mg/d in single or divided doses Ultramicrosize: 330–375 mg/d in single or divided doses Duration based on indication	NA	Microsize: [C: 125, 250] [S: 125 mg/5 mL] [T: 250, 500] Ultramicrosize: [T: 125, 165, 250, 330]
Itraconazole (*Sporanox*)	L	po: 200–400 mg/d; doses > 200 mg/d should be divided. Life-threatening infections: loading dose: 200 mg tid (600 mg/d) should be given for the first 3 d of therapy	NA	[C: 100] [S: 100 mg/10 mL]
Ketoconazole (*Nizoral*)	L, F	po: 200–400 mg qd Shampoo: 2/wk × 4 wk with at least 3 d between each shampoo Topical: apply qd–bid	NA	[Cream: 2%] [Shampoo: 2%] [T: 200]
Miconazole (*Monistat IV*)	L, F	IT: 20 mg q 1–2 d IV: initial: 200 mg, then 1.2–3.6 g/d divided q 8 h for up to 2 wk	NA	[Inj]

Note: NA = not applicable.
* The CrCl listed is the threshold below which the dose or frequency should be adjusted. See alternative reference or the drug package insert for detailed dosing guidelines.
** Adjust dose if decreased renal function is due to the drug, or give every other day.

MALNUTRITION

DEFINITION
There is no uniformly accepted definition of malnutrition in older persons. Some commonly used definitions include the following:

Community-Dwelling Men and Women
- Involuntary weight loss (eg, $\geq$ 10 lb over 6 months, $\geq$ 4% over 1 yr)
- Abnormal body mass index (eg, BMI > 27; BMI < 22)
- Hypoalbuminemia (eg, $\leq$ 3.8 g/dL)
- Hypocholesterolemia (eg, < 160 mg/dL)
- Specific vitamin or micronutrient deficiencies (eg, vitamin B_{12})

Hospitalized Patients
- Dietary intake (eg, < 50% of estimated needed caloric intake)
- Hypoalbuminemia (eg, < 3.5 g/dL)
- Hypocholesterolemia (eg, < 160 mg/dL)

Nursing-Home Patients (Triggered by the Minimum Data Set)
- Weight loss of $\geq$ 5% in past 30 d; $\geq$ 10% in 180 d
- Dietary intake of < 75% at most meals

EVALUATION
Multidimensional Assessment
In the absence of valid nutrition screening instruments, clinicians should focus on whether the following issues may be affecting nutritional status:
- Economic barriers to securing food
- Availability of sufficiently high-quality food
- Dental problems that prohibit ingesting high-quality food
- Medical illnesses that
  - interfere with digestion or absorption of food
  - increase nutritional requirements
  - require dietary restrictions (eg, low-sodium diet or npo)
- Functional disability that interferes with shopping, preparing meals, or feeding
- Food preferences or cultural beliefs that interfere with adequate food intake
- Poor appetite
- Depressive symptoms

Anthropometrics
Weight on each visit and yearly height (see p 1)

Biochemical Markers

Serum Proteins: All may drop precipitously because of trauma, sepsis, or major infection.
- Albumin (half-life 18–20 d) has prognostic value in all settings.
- Transferrin (half-life 7 d)
- Prealbumin (half-life 48 h) may be valuable in monitoring nutritional recovery.

Serum Cholesterol (Low or Falling Levels): Has prognostic value in all settings but may not be nutritionally mediated.

MANAGEMENT
Calculating Basic Energy (Caloric) and Fluid Requirements
- WHO energy estimates for adults aged 60 y and older:
  - Women (10.5) (weight in kg) + 596
  - Men (13.5) (weight in kg) + 487
- Harris-Benedict energy requirement equations:
  - Women 655 + (9.6) (weight in kg) + (1.7) (height in cm) − (4.7) (age in yr)
  - Men 66 + (13.7) (weight in kg) + (5.0) (height in cm) − (6.8) (age in yr)

Depending on activity and physiologic stress levels, these basic requirements may need to be increased (eg, 25% for sedentary or mild, 50% for moderate, and 100% for intense or severe activity or stress).
- Fluid requirements for older persons without cardiac or renal disease are approximately 30 mL/kg of body weight/d.

Oral and Enteral Formulas
Many formulas are available (see **Table 49**). Read the content labels and choose on the basis of calories/mL, protein, fiber, lactose, and fluid load.
- Oral: Many (eg, *Carnation Instant Breakfast, Health Shake*) are milk-based and provide approximately 1.0–1.5 calories/mL.
- Enteral: Commercial preparations have between 0.5 and 2.0 calories/mL; most contain no milk (lactose) products. For patients who need fluid restriction, the higher concentrated formulas may be valuable, but they may cause diarrhea. Because of reduced kidney function with aging, some recommend that protein should contribute no more than 20% of the formula's total calories. If formula is sole source of nutrition, consider one that contains fiber (25 g/d is optimal).

Table 49. Examples of Lactose-Free Oral and Enteral Products							
Product	Kcal/mL	mOsm	Protein (g/L)	Water (mL/L)	Na (mEq/L)	K (mEq/L)	Fiber (g/L)
Oral—low residue							
Boost Basic* (formerly Sustacal)	1.06	650	37.0	850	37.0	41.0	0
Boost Plus (formerly Sustacal)	1.50	670	61.0	780	37.0	38.0	< 4.0
Ensure*	1.06	470	37.3	845	37.0	40.0	0
Ensure Plus	1.50	690	54.9	769	46.0	40.0	0
Nu Basics	1.00	480	35.0	842	38.0	32.0	0
Nu Basics Plus	1.50	620	42.4	776	50.8	48.0	0
Oral—clear liquid							
Citrisource	0.76	700	37.0	876	10.0	1.6	0
Resource	1.06	430	33.0	842	24.0	1.3	0
Diabetes formulations							
Choicedm liquid	1.06	300–400	45.0	850	37.0	47.0	14.4
Glucerna	1.00	355	41.8	853	40.0	40.0	14.4
Enteral—low residue							
Isocal	1.06	270	34.0	850	23.0	34.0	0
Osmolite	1.06	300	37.2	841	28.0	26.0	0
Nutren 1.0	1.00	315	40.0	852	38.1	32.0	0
Enteral—low volume							
Deliver	2.00	640	75.0	710	35.0	43.0	0
Nutren 2.0	2.00	745	80.0	700	56.5	49.2	0
Enteral—high fiber							
Jevity	1.06	310	44.4	830	40.0	40.0	14.4
Ultracal	1.06	310	44.0	850	40.0	41.0	14.4
Nutren 1.0 with fiber	1.00	320	40.0	840	38.1	32.0	14.0

* Also has "pudding" and "with fiber" products that are similar. Fiber content: Boost Pudding, 0; Ensure Pudding, 0; Boost with Fiber, 11 g/L; Ensure Fiber with FOS, 12 g/L.

Important Drug-Enteral Interactions
- Soybean formulas increase fecal elimination of thyroxine; time administration of thyroxin and enteral nutrition as far apart as possible.
- Enteral feedings reduce absorption of phenytoin; administer phenytoin at least 2 h following a feeding and delay feeding at least 2 h after phenytoin is administered; monitor levels and adjust doses, as necessary.
- Check with pharmacy about suitability and best way to administer sustained-release, enteric-coated, and micro-encapsulated products (eg, omeprazole, lansoprazole, diltiazem, fluoxetine, verapamil).

Tips for Successful Tube Feeding
- Gastrostomy tube feeding may be either intermittent or continuous.
- Jejunostomy tube feedings must be continuous.
- Continuous tube feeding is associated with less frequent diarrhea but with higher rates of tube clogging.

- To prevent clogging and to provide additional free water, flushing with at least 30–60 cc of water 4–6 times a day is recommended. Sometimes sugar-free carbonated beverages, cranberry juice, or meat tenderizer can restore patency to clogged tubes.
- Diarrhea, which occurs in 5%–30% of persons receiving enteral feeding, may be related to the osmolality of the formula, the rate of delivery, high sorbitol content in liquid medications (eg, acetaminophen, lithium, oxybutynin, furosemide), or other patient-related factors such as antibiotic use or impaired absorption.
- To help prevent aspiration, maintain a 30-degree elevation of the head of the bed during continuous feeding and for at least 2 h following bolus feedings.
- Do not administer bulk-forming laxatives (eg, methylcellulose or psyllium) through feeding tubes.
- Check gastric residual volume before each bolus feeding and hold feeding for at least 1 h if residual is more than half of previous feeding volume. Metoclopramide (*Reglan*) 5–10 mg [5 mg/5 mL] qid may be useful for high gastric residual volume problems once mechanical obstruction has been excluded.

Parenteral Nutrition
Indicated in those with digestive dysfunction precluding enteral feeding. Delivers protein as amino acids, carbohydrate as dextrose, and fat as lipid emulsions.
Peripheral Parenteral Nutrition: Requires rotation of peripheral IV site every 72 h. Solution osmolarity of less than 900 mOsm/L is recommended to reduce risk of phlebitis (see **Table 50**).
Total Parenteral Nutrition: Must be administered through a central catheter, which may be inserted peripherally.

Table 50. Caloric Value and Osmolarity of Parenteral Solutions		
Resolution	**Caloric Value (Kcal/L)**	**Osmolarity (mOsm/L)**
Dextrose (%)		
5	170	250
10	340	500
20	680	1000
Lipid emulsions (%)		
10	1100	230
20	2200	330–340

Source: Bçikston SJ. In: Ewald GA, McKenzie CR. *Manual of Medical Therapeutics.* 28th ed. Boston: Little, Brown; 1995:36. Copyright © 1995 by Little, Brown & Company. Reprinted with permission.

SHOULDER PAIN: DIFFERENTIAL DIAGNOSIS AND DISTINGUISHING FEATURES

Rotator Cuff Tendinitis, Subacromial Bursitis, or Rotator Tendon Impingement on Clavicle

Dull ache radiating to upper arm. Painful arc (on abduction 60–120 degrees and external rotation) is characteristic. Also can be distinguished by applying resistance against active range of motion while immobilizing the neck with hand.

Treatment: Identify and eliminate provocative, repetitive injury (eg, avoid overhead reaching). A brief period of rest and immobilization with a sling may be helpful. Pain control with acetaminophen or NSAIDs **(Table 51)**, home exercises or PT (especially assisted range of motion and wall walking), and corticosteroid injections may be useful.

Rotator Cuff Tears

Mild to complete; characterized by diminished shoulder movement. If severe, patients do not have full range of active or passive motion. The "drop arm" sign (the inability to maintain the arm in an abducted 90-degree position) indicates supraspinatus and infraspinatus tear. Weakness of external rotation (elbows flexed, thumbs up with examiner's hands outside patient's elbows; patient is asked to resist inward pressure) is common. MRI establishes diagnosis.

Treatment: If due to injury, a brief period of rest and immobilization with a sling may be helpful. Pain control with acetaminophen or NSAIDs **(Table 51)**, home exercises or PT (especially assisted range of motion and wall walking) may be useful. If no improvement after 6–8 wk of conservative measures, consider surgical repair.

Bicipital Tendinitis

Pain felt on anterior lateral aspect of shoulder, tenderness in the groove between greater and lesser tuberosities of the humerus. Pain is produced on resisted flexion of shoulder, flexion of the elbow, or supination (external rotation) of the hand and wrist with the elbow flexed at the side.

Treatment: Identify and eliminate provocative, repetitive activities (eg, avoid overhead reaching). A period of rest (at least 7 d with no lifting) and corticosteroid injections are major components of therapy. After rest period, PT should focus on stretching biceps tendon (eg, putting arm on doorframe and hyperextending shoulder, with some external rotation).

Frozen Shoulder (Adhesive Capsulitis)

Loss of passive external (lateral) rotation, abduction, and internal rotation of the shoulder to less than 90 degrees. Usually follows three phases: painful (freezing) phase lasting wks to a few mo; adhesive (stiffening) phase lasting 4–12 mo; resolution phase lasting 6–24 mo.

Treatment: Avoid rest and begin PT and home exercises for stretching the arm in flexion, horizontal adduction, and internal and external rotation. Corticosteroid injections may reduce pain and permit more aggressive PT. Consider surgical manipulation under anesthesia or arthroscopic dilation of capsule.

BACK PAIN: DIFFERENTIAL DIAGNOSIS AND DISTINGUISHING FEATURES

Acute Lumbar Strain (Low Back Pain Syndrome)

Acute pain frequently precipitated by heavy lifting or exercise. Pain may be central or more prominent on one side and may radiate to sacroiliac region and buttocks. Pain is aggravated by motion, standing, and prolonged sitting, and relieved by rest. Sciatic pain may be present even when neurologic examination is normal.

Treatment: Most can continue normal activities. If a patient obtains symptomatic relief from bed rest, generally 1–2 d lying in a semi-Fowler position or on side with the hips and knees flexed with pillow between legs will suffice. Treat muscle spasm with the application of ice, preferably in a massage over the muscles in spasm. Acetaminophen or NSAIDs (**Table 51**) can be used to control pain. As pain diminishes, encourage patient to begin isometric abdominal and lower-extremity exercises. Symptoms often recur. Education on back posture, lifting precautions, and abdominal muscle strengthening may help prevent recurrences.

Acute Disk Herniation

Over 90% of cases occur at L4–L5 or L5–S1 levels, resulting in unilateral impairment of ankle reflex, toe and ankle dorsiflexion, and pain (commonly sciatic) on straight leg raising (can be tested from sitting position by leg extension). Pain is acute in onset and varies considerably with changes in position.

Treatment: Initially same as acute lumbar strain (above). If unresponsive, administer epidural injection of a combination of a long-acting corticosteroid with an epidural anesthetic. Consider surgery if recurrence or persistence with neurologic signs beyond 6–8 wk after conservative treatment. The value of epidural injections and surgery for pain without neurologic signs is controversial. (See **Table 2** and **Table 3**.)

Osteoarthritis and Chronic Disk Degeneration

Characterized by aching pain aggravated by motion and relieved by rest. Occasionally, hypertrophic spurring in a facet joint may cause unilateral radiculopathy with sciatica.

Treatment: Identify and eliminate provocative activities. Education on back posture, lifting precautions, and abdominal muscle strengthening. Acetaminophen or NSAIDs (**Table 51**). Corticosteroid injections may be useful. Consider opioids and other pain treatment modalities for chronic refractory pain (see p 108).

Unstable Lumbar Spine

Severe, sudden, short-lasting, frequently recurrent pain often brought on by sudden, unguarded movements. Pain is reproduced upon moving from the flexed to the erect position. Pain is usually relieved by lying supine or on side. Impingement on nerve roots by spurs from facet joints or herniated disks can cause similar complaints, although symptoms in these conditions usually worsen as time passes. Symptoms can mimic disk herniation or degeneration, or osteoarthritis. Lumbar flexion x-rays can be diagnostic.

Lumbar Spinal Stenosis

Symptoms increase on spinal extension (eg, with prolonged standing, walking downhill, lying prone) and decrease with spinal flexion (eg, sitting, bending forward while walking, lying in the flexed position). Only symptom may be fatigue and/or pain in legs when walking (pseudo-claudication). May have immobility of lumbar spine, pain with straight leg raises, weakness of muscles innervated by L4 through S1 (see **Table 2**). Over 4 yr, 15% improve, 15% deteriorate, and 70% remain stable.

Treatment: Acetaminophen or NSAIDs (**Table 51**) and exercises to reduce lumbar lordosis are sometimes beneficial. Corticosteroid injections may be useful. Surgical intervention is more effective than conservative treatment in relieving moderate or severe symptoms; however, recurrence of pain several years after surgery is common.

Vertebral Compression Fracture
Immediate onset of severe pain; worse with sitting or standing; sometimes relieved by lying down.

Treatment: See Osteoporosis (p 105). Bed rest, analgesia, and mobilization as tolerated. Calcitonin may provide symptomatic improvement. May require hospitalization to control symptoms. Percutaneous vertebroplasty or kyphoplasty may be effective for pain relief in refractory cases, but clinical trial data are lacking.

Nonrheumatic Pain (eg, Tumors, Aneurysms)
Gradual onset, steadily expanding, often unrelated to position and not relieved by lying down. Night pain when lying down is characteristic. Upper motor neuron signs may be present. Involvement is usually in thoracic and upper lumbar spine.

HIP PAIN: DIFFERENTIAL DIAGNOSIS AND DISTINGUISHING FEATURES
Trochanteric Bursitis
Pain in lateral aspect of the hip that usually worsens when patient sits on a hard chair, lies on the affected side, or rises from a chair or bed; pain may improve with walking. Local tenderness over greater trochanter is often present, and pain is often reproduced on resisted abduction of the leg or internal rotation of the hip. However, trochanteric bursitis does not produce limited range of motion, pain on range of motion, pain in the groin, or radicular signs.

Treatment: Identify and eliminate provocative activities. Check for leg length discrepancy, prescribe orthotics if appropriate. Injection of a combination of a long-acting corticosteroid with an anesthetic is most effective treatment.

Osteoarthritis
"Boring" quality pain in the hip, often in the groin, and sometimes referred to the back or knee with stiffness after rest. Passive motion is restricted in all directions if disease is fairly advanced. In early disease, pain in the groin on internal rotation of the hip is characteristic.

Treatment: See Osteoarthritis (p 91). Elective total hip replacement is indicated for patients who have radiographic evidence of joint damage and moderate to severe persistent pain or disability, or both, that is not substantially relieved by an extended course of nonsurgical management.

National Institutes of Health Consensus Development Conference Statement September 12–14, 1994 (reviewed 1998).

Hip Fracture
Sudden onset, usually after a fall, with inability to walk or bear weight, frequently radiating to groin or knee.

Treatment: Treatment is surgical with open reduction and internal fixation, hemiarthroplasty, or total hip replacement, depending on site of fracture and amount of displacement. For patients who were nonambulatory prior to the fracture, conservative management is an option.

Nonrheumatic Pain

Referred pain from viscera, radicular pain from the lower spine, avascular necrosis, Paget's disease, metastasis.

OSTEOARTHRITIS
Nonpharmacologic Approaches

- Superficial heat: Hot packs, heating pads, paraffin, or hot water bottles (moist heat is better).
- Deep heat: Microwave, shortwave diathermy, or ultrasound.
- Biofeedback and transcutaneous electrical nerve stimulation.
- Exercise (especially water-based), PT, OT: Strengthening, stretching, range of motion, functional activities.
- Weight loss: Especially for low back, hip, and knee arthritis.
- Splinting: Avoid splinting for long periods of time (eg, > 6 wk) since periarticular muscle weakness and wasting may occur.
- Assistive devices: Cane should be used in the hand contralateral to the affected knee or hip.
- Surgical intervention (eg, debridement, meniscal repair, prosthetic joint replacement).

Pharmacologic Intervention (See also p 108.)
Topical Analgesics: Liniment, capsaicin cream.
Intra-articular Injections:

- Corticosteroids: May be particularly effective if monoarticular symptoms (eg, methylprednisolone acetate, triamcinolone acetonide, and triamcinolone hexacetonide) 20–40 mg for large joints (eg, knee, ankle, shoulder), 10–20 mg for wrists and elbows, and 5–15 mg for small joints of hands and feet; often mixed with lidocaine 1% or its equivalent (in equal volume with corticosteroids) for immediate relief.
- Hyaluronan: Sodium hyaluronate (*Hyalgan*) injections weekly for 5 wk or hylan G-F 20 (*Synvisc*) 3 injections 1 wk apart for knee osteoarthritis.

Initial Drug Treatment of Choice: Acetaminophen not to exceed 4 g/d (ACR) (see **Table 51**).

NSAIDs: Often provide pain relief but have higher rates of side effects (see **Table 51**). Misoprostol (*Cytotec*) 100–200 mg qid with food [T: 100, 200] or a proton-pump inhibitor (see **Table 32**) may be valuable prophylaxis against NSAID-induced ulcers in high-risk patients. Selective COX-2 inhibitors have lower likelihood of causing gastroduodenal ulcers than nonselective NSAIDs. All may increase INR in patients receiving wafarin.

Oral Analgesics: Eg, tramadol, other opioids (see **Table 61**).

Table 51. Acetaminophen and Nonsteroidal Anti-Inflammatory Drugs

Class, Drug	Usual Dosage for Arthritis	Formulations	Comments (Metabolism, Excretion)
Acetaminophen (*Tylenol*)	650 mg q 4–6 h	[T: 80, 325, 500, 650; caplet: 160, 325, 500; elixir: 120/5 mL, 160/5 mL, 167/5 mL, 325/5 mL; S: 160/5 mL, 500/15 mL; Sp: 120, 325, 600]	Drug of choice for chronic musculoskeletal conditions; no anti-inflammatory properties; hepatotoxic above 4 g/d; at high doses (≥ 2g/d) may increase INR in patients receiving warfarin (L, K)
(*Tylenol ER*)	1300 mg tid	[ER: 650]	
Aspirin	650 mg q 4–6 h	[81, 325, 500, 650, 975; Sp: 120, 200, 300, 600]	(K)
Extended release (*Ext Release Bayer 8 Hour,* ZORprin*)	1300 mg tid or 1600–3200 mg bid	[CR: 650, 800]	
Enteric-coated*	1000 mg qid		
Nonacetylated Salicylates			Do not inhibit platelet aggregation; fewer GI and renal side effects; no reaction in ASA-sensitive patients
Choline magnesium salicylate (*Tricosal, Trilisate*)	3 g/d in 1, 2, or 3 doses	[T: 500, 750, 1000; S: 500 mg/mL]	(K)
Choline salicylate (*Arthropan*)	4.8–7.2 g/d divided	[S: 870 mg/5 mL]	(L, K)
Magnesium salicylate (*Doan's, Magan, Mobidin*)	650–1090 mg tid–qid	[T: 325, 467, 500, 545, 587, 600, 650]	Avoid in renal failure
Salicylsalicylic acid (salsalate) (eg, *Disalcid, Mono-Gesic, Salflex*)	1500 mg to 4 g/d in 2 or 3 doses	[T: 500, 750; C: 500]	(K)
Sodium salicylate*	3.6–5.4 g/d divided	[T: 325, 650]	
Nonselective NSAIDs			
Diclofenac (*Cataflam, Voltaren*)	50–150 mg/d in 2 or 3 doses	[T: 25, 50, 75, 100]	(L)

Table 51. Acetaminophen and Nonsteroidal Anti-Inflammatory Drugs (cont.)			
Class, Drug	Usual Dosage for Arthritis	Formulations	Comments (Metabolism, Excretion)
Extended release 50 mg with 200 µg misoprostol (*Arthrotec 50*) 75 mg with 200 µg misoprostol (*Arthrotec 75*)	100 mg/d	[T: 100]	(L)
Diflunisal (*Dolobid*)	500–1000 mg/d in 2 doses	[T: 250, 500]	(K)
Etodolac (*Lodine*)	200–400 mg tid–qid	[T: 400, 500; ER 400, 500, 600; C: 200, 300]	Fewer GI side effects (L)
Fenoprofen (*Nalfon*)	200–600 mg tid–qid	[C: 200, 300; T: 600]	Higher risk of GI side effects (L)
Flurbiprofen (*Ansaid*)	200–300 mg/d in 2, 3, or 4 doses	[T: 50, 100]	(L)
Ibuprofen (eg, *Advil, Motrin, Nuprin*)**	1200–3200 mg/d in 3 or 4 doses	[T: 100, 200, 400, 600, 800; CT: 50, 100; S: 100 mg/5 mL]	Fewer GI side effects (L)
Indomethacin (*Indochron, Indocin*)	25–50 mg bid–tid	[C: 25, 50; Sp: 50; S: 25 mg/5 mL]	High risk of GI side effects; increased risk of CNS side effects (L)
Extended release (*Indocin SR*)	75 mg/d or bid	[T: 75]	Increased risk of CNS side effects
Ketoprofen (*Actron, Orudis*)	50–75 mg tid	[T: 12.5; C: 25, 50, 75]	(L)
Sustained release (*Oruvail*)	200 mg/d	[C: 100, 150, 200]	(L)
Ketorolac (*Toradol*)	10 mg q 4–6 h, 15 mg IM or IV q 6 h	[T: 10; Inj]	Duration of use should be limited to 5 d (K)
Meclofenamate sodium	200–400 mg/d in 3 or 4 doses	[C: 50, 100]	High incidence of diarrhea (L)
Meloxicam (*Mobic*)	7.5–15 mg/d	[T: 7.5, 15]	Has some COX-2 selectivity (L)
Nabumetone (*Relafen*)	500–1000 mg bid	[T: 500, 750]	Fewer GI side effects (L)
Naproxen (*Aleve,*** *Naprosyn*)	200–500 mg bid–tid	[T: 200, 250, 375, 500; S: 125 mg/5 mL]	(L)
Delayed release (*EC-Naprosyn*)	375–500 mg bid	[T: 375, 500]	(L)

(continues)

Class, Drug	Usual Dosage for Arthritis	Formulations	Comments (Metabolism, Excretion)
Controlled release (*Naprelan*)	750–1000 mg daily	[T: 375, 500, 750]	(L)
Naproxen sodium (*Anaprox*)	275 mg or 550 mg bid	[T: 275, 550]	
Oxaprozin (*Daypro*)	1200 mg/d	[C: 600]	(L)
Piroxicam (*Feldene*)	10 mg/d	[T: 10, 20]	(L)
Sulindac (*Clinoril*)	150–200 mg bid	[T: 150, 200]	May have higher rate of renal impairment (L)
Tolmetin (*Tolectin*)	600–1800 mg/d in 3 or 4 doses	[T: 200, 600; C: 400]	(L)
Selective COX-2 Inhibitors			Less GI ulceration; do not inhibit platelets
Celecoxib (*Celebrex*)	100–200 mg bid	[C: 100, 200]	Contraindicated if allergic to sulfonamides; may increase INR if taking warfarin; avoid if moderate or severe hepatic insufficiency
Rofecoxib (*Vioxx*)	12.5–25 once daily	[T: 12.5, 25, 50; S: 12.5 mg/5 mL, 25 mg/5 mL]	May increase INR if taking warfarin; avoid if moderate or severe hepatic insufficiency

* Also available without prescription in a lower tablet strength.
** Available without a prescription.

GOUT
Definition
Urate crystal disease that may be expressed as acute gouty arthritis, usually in a single joint of foot, ankle, knee, or olecranon bursa; or chronic arthritis.

Precipitating Factors
- Alcohol, heavy ingestion
- Allopurinol, stopping or starting
- Binge eating
- Dehydration
- Diuretics
- Fasting
- Infection
- Serum uric acid levels, any change up or down
- Surgery

Evaluation of Acute Gouty Arthritis
Joint aspiration to remove crystals and microscopic examination to establish diagnosis; serum uric acid (can be normal during flare).

Management

Treatment of Acute Gouty Flare: Experts differ regarding order of choices:

- Intra-articular injections (see p 91)
- NSAIDs (see **Table 51**)
- Colchicine (more toxic in older persons; more effective if given within 24 hr of symptom onset)
  - Oral 0.5–0.6 mg (1 tablet) q 1–2 h until symptoms abate, GI toxicity occurs, or maximum dose of 6 mg/24-h period has been given.
  - IV 1–2 mg in 10–20 mL NS given over 3–5 min
    - may repeat the following day
    - contraindicated in patients who have had recent oral colchicine
    - avoid in patients with renal or hepatic disease
    - potential for severe bone marrow toxicity
- Prednisone 20–40 mg po qd until response, then rapid taper
- ACTH 75 IU SC or cosyntropin (*Cortrosyn*) 75 µg SC; may repeat daily for 3 d

Treatment of Hyperuricemia Following Acute Flare: Colchicine 0.5–0.6 mg/d for 2–4 wk prior to initiation of any treatment in **Table 52** and continued until serum uric acid has returned to normal.

Table 52. Medications Useful in Managing Chronic Gout			
Drug	**Usual Dosage**	**Formulations**	**Comments (Metabolism, Excretion)**
Allopurinol (*Zyloprim*)	100–200 mg qd	[T: 100, 300]	Do not initiate during flare; reduce dose in renal or hepatic impairment; increase dose by 100 mg every 2–4 wk to normalize serum urate level; monitor CBC; rash is common (K)
Colchicine	0.5–0.6 mg	[T: 0.5, 0.6]	Follow CBC (L)
Probenecid (*Benemid*)	500–1500 mg in 2–3 divided doses	[T: 500]	Adjust dose to normalize serum urate level or increase urine urate excretion; inhibits platelet function; may not be effective if renal impairment (K, L)
Sulfinpyrazone (*Anturane*)	50 mg po bid to 100 mg qid	[T: 100, 200; C: 200]	Inhibits platelet function (K)

PSEUDOGOUT

Definition

Crystal-induced arthritis (especially affecting wrists and knees) associated with calcium pyrophosphate.

Risk Factors

- Advanced osteoarthritis
- Diabetes mellitus
- Gout
- Hemochromatosis
- Hypercalcemia
- Hyperparathyroidism
- Hypomagnesemia
- Hypophosphatemia
- Hypothyroidism
- Neuropathic joints
- Older age

Precipitating Factors
• Acute illness   • Dehydration   • Minor trauma   • Surgery

Evaluation of Acute Arthritis
Joint aspiration and microscopic examination to establish diagnosis; x-ray indicating chondrocalcinosis (best seen in wrists, knees, shoulder, symphysis pubis).

Management of Acute Flare
See **Gout** (p 95). Colchicine is less effective.

POLYMYALGIA RHEUMATICA, GIANT CELL (TEMPORAL) ARTERITIS
Definitions
Polymyalgia Rheumatica (PMR): proximal limb and girdle stiffness without tenderness but with constitutional symptoms (eg, fatigue, malaise) and elevated sedimentation rate, often ≥ 100.
Giant Cell (Temporal) Arteritis (GCA): medium to large vessel vasculitis that presents with symptoms of PMR, headache, scalp tenderness, jaw or tongue claudication, visual disturbances, TIA or stroke, and elevated sedimentation rate.

Diagnosis and Management
• PMR is a clinical diagnosis supported by an increased sedimentation rate. Management is low-dose (eg, 5–20 mg/d) prednisone or its equivalent. Some patients with milder symptoms may respond to NSAIDs alone. Follow symptoms and sedimentation rate. Maintain therapy for at least 1 yr to prevent relapse. Consider osteoporosis prevention medication (see p 105).
• GCA is confirmed by temporal artery biopsy, but treatment should not wait for pathologic diagnosis. Begin prednisone (1.0–1.5 mg/kg/d) or its equivalent while biopsy and pathology are pending. Taper to lowest dose that will control symptoms and sedimentation rate. Maintain therapy for at least 1 yr to prevent relapse. Consider osteoporosis prevention medication (see p 105).

NEUROLOGIC DISORDERS

TREMORS

Table 53. Classification of Tremors				
Type	Hz	Associated Conditions	Features	Treatment
Cerebellar	3–5	Cerebellar disease	Present only during movement; ↑ with intention; ↑ amplitude as target is approached	Symptomatic management
Essential	6–12	Familial in 50% of cases	Varying amplitude; common in upper extremities, head, neck; ↑ with anti-gravity movements, intention, stress, medications	Long-acting propranolol (see p 28); or primidone (*Mysoline*) 100 mg qhs start, titrate to 0.5–1.0 g/d in 3–4 divided doses [T: 50, 250; S: 250 mg/5 mL]
Parkinson's	3–7	Parkinson's disease, parkinsonism	"Pill rolling;" present at rest; ↑ with emotional stress or when examiner calls attention to it; commonly asymmetric	See Parkinson's disease (p 100)
Physiologic	8–12	Normal	Low amplitude; ↑ with stress, anxiety, emotional upset, lack of sleep, fatigue, toxins, medications	Treatment of exacerbating factor

DIZZINESS

Table 54. Classification of Dizziness				
Primary Symptom	Features	Duration	Diagnosis	Management
Dizziness	Lightheadedness 1–30 min after standing	Seconds to minutes (E)	Orthostatic hypotension	See p 57
	Impairment in > 1 of the following: vision, vestibular function, spinal proprioception, cerebellum, lower-extremity peripheral nerves	Occurs with ambulation (C)	Multiple sensory impairments	Correct or maximize sensory deficits; PT for balance and strength training
	Unsteady gait with short steps; ↑ reflexes and/or tone	Occurs with ambulation (C)	Ischemic cerebral disease	Aspirin; modification of vascular risk factors; PT

(continues)

Primary Symptom	Features	Duration	Diagnosis	Management
	Provoked by head or neck movement; reduced neck range of motion	Seconds to minutes (E)	Cervical spondylosis	Behavior modification; reduce cervical spasm and inflammation
Drop attacks	Provoked by head or neck movement, reduced vertebral artery flow seen on Doppler or angiography	Seconds to minutes (E)	Postural impingement of vertebral artery	Behavior modification
Vertigo	Brought on by position change, positive Dix-Hallpike test	Seconds to minutes (E)	Benign paroxysmal positional vertigo	Epley's maneuvers to reposition crystalline debris; exercises provoking symptoms may be of help
	Vascular disease risk factors, cranial nerve abnormalities	10 min to several hours (E)	Transient ischemic attacks	Aspirin; modification of vascular risk factors

Note: C = chronic; E = episodic.
Source: Data from Colledge NR, Barr-Hamilton RM, Lewis SJ, et al. Evaluation of investigations to diagnose the causes of dizziness in elderly people: a community based controlled study. *BMJ.* 1996;313(7060):788–792.

MANAGEMENT OF ACUTE STROKE
Attempt to Diagnose Cause
Examination:
- Cardiac (murmurs, arrhythmias, enlargement)
- Neurologic (serial examinations)
- Optic fundi
- Vascular (carotids and other peripheral pulses)

Tests:
• ABG	• BUN	• Creatinine	• Electrolytes
• Brain imaging (CT is adequate)	• CBC	• ECG	• ESR
	• LFTs		

Transesophageal echocardiography is preferred over transthoracic echocardiography for detection of cardiogenic emboli. Carotid duplex and transcranial Doppler studies can detect carotid and vertebrobasilar embolic sources, respectively. Magnetic resonance angiography is indicated if one is considering emergent thrombolytic therapy to reverse stroke progression (thrombolytic therapy is of unproven benefit in older adults).

Provide Supportive Care
- Control BP: Do not lower SBP if it is < 180; higher BP should be lowered *gently*; some experts recommend not lowering SBP unless it is > 200.
- Correct metabolic imbalances.
- Monitor and treat for hypoxia.
- Monitor for depression.
- Refer to rehabilitation when medically stable.

Halt or Reverse Progression

Acute Noncardioembolic Stroke or TIA: Use aspirin, 325 mg/d (range 81–1300 mg/d) or low-dose SC heparin, or both. The benefit of emergent thrombolytic therapy is unproven in older adults and should be considered on a case-by-case basis.

Cardioembolic Stroke: Begin full-dose heparin or warfarin anticoagulation starting day 3–7; timing of anticoagulation depends on size of infarct. (See also p 14.)

Progressing Stroke or Crescendo TIAs: Even though there is no evidence that anticoagulation improves outcomes, some clinicians recommend it in this situation; aspirin would be more conservative therapy.

Hemorrhagic Stroke: Supportive care.

STROKE PREVENTION
Risk Factor Modification
- Stop smoking
- Reduce SBP (goal < 140 mm Hg)
- Lower serum LDL (goal < 130 mg/dL)
- Start anticoagulation or antiplatelet therapy for atrial fibrillation (see p 14)

Antiplatelet Therapy for Patients With Prior TIA or Stroke
- First line is acetylsalicylic acid (ASA) 325 mg qd.
- Clopidogrel (*Plavix*) 75 mg qd [T: 75] if intolerant to ASA or aspirin failure.
- Ticlopidine (*Ticlid*) 250 mg bid [T: 250] requires regular blood monitoring.
- Addition of dipyridamole (*Persantine*) 200–400 mg/d [T: 25, 50, 75] in divided doses to ASA may provide additional benefit. A combination form of aspirin (25 mg) and dipyridamole (200 mg) (*Aggrenox*) 1 tablet bid is now available.
- Efficacy of warfarin therapy in the absence of atrial fibrillation is unproven.

Table 55. Treatment Options for Carotid Stenosis			
Presentation	**% Stenosis**	**Preferred Rχ**	**Comments**
Prior TIA or stroke	≥ 70	CE	CE superior to medical therapy only if patient is reasonable surgical risk and facility has track record of low complication rate for CE (<5%)
Prior TIA or stroke	50–69	CE or MM	Serial carotid Doppler testing may identify rapidly developing plaques
Prior TIA or stroke	< 50	MM	CE of no proven benefit in this situation
Asymptomatic	≥ 80	CE or MM	CE should be considered only for the most healthy
Asymptomatic	< 80	MM	CE of no proven benefit in this situation

Note: CE = carotid endarterectomy; MM = medical management.

PARKINSON'S DISEASE

Parkinson's Disease Diagnosis Requires:

Bradykinesia, eg,

- Slowness of initiation of voluntary movements (eg, glue-footedness during gait initiation)
- Reduced speed and amplitude of repetitive movements (eg, tapping index finger and thumb together)
- Difficulty switching from one motor program to another (eg, multiple steps to turn during gait testing)

and 1 or more of the following:

- Muscular rigidity (eg, cogwheeling)
- 4–6 Hz resting tremor
- Impaired righting reflex (eg, retropulsed during sternal nudge)

Nonpharmacologic Management

- Patient education is essential, and support groups are often helpful; see p 230 for telephone numbers, Web sites.
- Exercise program
- Surgical therapies can be considered for disabling symptoms refractory to medical therapy. Tremor can be improved by thalamotomy or thalamic stimulation (fewer side effects). Dyskinesias can be treated by pallidotomy or pallidal and subthalamic stimulation.

Table 56. Drugs for Parkinson's Disease			
Class, Drug	**Initial Dosage**	**Formu- lations**	**Comments (Metabolism, Excretion)**
Anticholinergics			
Benztropine (*Cogentin*)	0.5 mg po qd	[T: 0.5, 1, 2]	Can cause confusion and delirium; helpful for drooling (L, K)
Trihexyphenidyl (*Artane, Trihexy*)	1 mg qd	[T: 2, 5; S: 2 mg/5 mL]	Same as above (L, K)
Dopamine			
Levodopa-carbidopa (*Sinemet*)	1 tab tid	[T: 10/100, 25/100, 25/250]	Mainstay of PD therapy; increase dose as needed; watch for GI side effects, orthostatic hypotension, confusion (L)
Slow-release levodopa-carbidopa (*Sinemet CR*)	1 tab bid	[T: 25/100, 50/200]	Useful at daily dopamine requirement ≥ 300 mg/d; slower absorption than carbidopa-levodopa; can improve motor fluctuations (L)
Dopamine agonists			
Bromocriptine (*Parlodel*)	1.25 mg bid	[T: 2.5; C: 5]	Titrate over 3–4 wk to effective dose (15–30 mg/d); very expensive (L)
Pergolide (*Permax*)	0.05 mg qd	[T: 0.05, 0.25, 1]	Titrate over 3–4 wk to effective dose (1–4 mg/d); very expensive (K)

Table 56. Drugs for Parkinson's Disease (cont.)			
Class, Drug	Initial Dosage	Formu-lations	Comments (Metabolism, Excretion)
Pramipexole (*Mirapex*)	0.125 mg tid	[T: 0.125, 0.25, 0.5, 1, 1.5]	Titrate over 3–4 wk to effective dose (1.5–4.5 mg/d) (K)
Ropinirole (*Requip*)	0.25 mg tid	[T: 0.25, 0.5, 1, 2, 5]	Titrate over 3–4 wk to effective dose (3–16 mg/d); appropriate as first-line drug in early PD (L)
Catechol *O*-methyl-transferase (COMT) inhibitor			
Tolcapone (*Tasmar*)	100 mg tid	[T: 100, 200]	Monitor LFT q 6 mo (L, K)
Entacapone (*Comtan*)	200 mg with each L-dopa dose	[T: 200]	Adjunctive therapy with L-dopa; watch for nausea, orthostatic hypotension (L)
Dopamine reuptake inhibitor			
Amantadine (*Symmetrel*)	100 mg qd–bid	[T: 100; C: 100; S: 50 mg/5 mL]	Useful in early and late PD; watch closely for CNS side effects; do not discontinue abruptly (K)
MAO B inhibitor			
Selegiline (*Carbex, Eldepryl*)	5 mg bid qam & noon	[T: 5]	Symptomatic benefit; not proven to be neuroprotective; expensive (L, K)

Note: PD = Parkinson's disease.

SEIZURES
Classification
- Generalized: All areas of brain affected with alteration in consciousness.
- Partial: Focal brain area affected, not necessarily with alteration in consciousness; can progress to generalized type.

Evaluation, Assessment
Initial:
- History: Neurologic disorders, trauma, drug and alcohol use
- Physical examination: General, with careful neurologic
- Routine tests: BUN, calcium, CBC, creatinine, ECG, EEG, electrolytes, glucose, head CT, LFT, magnesium
- Tests as indicated: Head MRI, lumbar puncture, oxygen saturation, urine toxic or drug screen

Common Causes:
- Advanced dementia
- CNS infection
- Drug or alcohol withdrawal
- Idiopathic causes
- Metabolic disorders
- Prior stroke (most common)
- Toxins
- Trauma
- Tumor

Management
- Treat underlying causes.
- Institute antiepileptic therapy (see **Table 57**). Virtually all antiepileptics can cause sedation and ataxia.

Table 57. Antiepileptic Therapy in Elderly Patients

Drug	Dosage (mg)	Target Blood Level (µg/mL)	Formulations	Comments (Metabolism, Excretion)
Carbamazepine (*Tegretol*)	200–600 bid	4–12	[T: 100, 200; S: 100/ 5 mL]	Many drug interactions; mood stabilizer; SR preparation (*Tegretol XR*) also available [T: 100, 200, 400; C: CR 200, 300] (L, K)
Gabapentin (*Neurontin*)	300–600 tid	NA	[C: 100, 300, 400; T: 600, 800; S: 250/ 5 mL]	Used as adjunct to other agents; adjust dose on basis of creatinine clearance (K)
Lamotrigine (*Lamictal*)	100–300 bid	2–4	[T: 25, 100, 150, 200]	When used with valproic acid, begin at 25 mg qd, titrate to 25–100 mg bid (L, K)
Oxcarbazepine (*Trileptal*)	300–1200 bid	NA	[T: 150, 300, 600]	Similar to carbamazepine; can rarely cause hyponatremia (L)
Phenobarbital (*Luminal*)	30–60 bid– tid	20–40	[T: 8, 15, 16, 30, 32, 60; S: 15/ 5 mL; 20/ 5 mL]	Many drug interactions; not recommended for use in elderly patients (L)
Phenytoin (*Dilantin*)	200–300 qd	5–20*	[C: 30, 100; CT: 50; S: 125/5 mL]	Many drug interactions (L)
Tiagabine (*Gabitril Filmtabs*)	2–12 bid–tid	NA	[T: 2, 4, 12, 16, 20]	Side-effect profile in elderly less well described (L)
Topiramate (*Topamax*)	25–100 qd–bid	NA	[T: 25, 100, 200; C: 15, 25]	May affect cognitive functioning at high doses (L, K)
Valproic acid (*Depacon*, *Depakene*, *Depakote*)	250–750 tid	50–100	[T: 125, 250, 500; C: 125, 250; S: 250/5 mL]	Can cause weight gain; several drug interactions; mood stabilizer; follow LFTs and platelets; SR preparation (*Depakote ER*) also available [T: 500] (L)

Note: NA = not available.
*Phenytoin is extensively bound to plasma albumin. In cases of hypoalbuminemia or marked renal insufficiency, calculate adjusted phenytoin concentration (C):

$$C_{adjusted} = \frac{C_{observed}\ (\mu g/mL)}{0.2 \times albumin\ (g/dL) + 0.1}.$$

If creatinine clearance < 10 mL/min, use:

$$C_{adjusted} = \frac{C_{observed}\ (\mu g/mL)}{0.1 \times albumin\ (gdL) + 0.1}.$$

Obtaining a free phenytoin level is an alternate method for monitoring phenytoin in cases of hypoalbuminemia or marked renal insufficiency.

APHASIA

Table 58. Aphasias in Which Repetition Is Impaired				
Type	Fluency	Auditory Comprehension	Associated Neurologic Deficits	Comments
Broca's	−	+	Right hemiparesis	Patient aware of deficit; high rate of associated depression; message board helpful for communication
Wernicke's	+	−	Often none	Patient frequently unaware of deficit; speech content usually unintelligible; therapy often focuses on visually based communication
Conduction	+	+	Occasional right facial weakness	Patient usually aware of the deficit; speech content usually intelligible
Global	−	−	Right hemiplegia with right field cut	Most commonly due to left middle cerebral artery thrombosis, which, if this is the cause, carries a poor prognosis for meaningful speech recovery

PERIPHERAL NEUROPATHY
Diagnosis See **Figure 4**.

Treatment
Prevention of Complications:
- Protect distal extremities from trauma—appropriate shoe size, daily foot inspections, good skin care, avoidance of barefoot walking.
- Maintain tight glycemic control in diabetic neuropathy.

Treatment of Painful Neuropathy: Start at low dose, increase as needed and tolerated:
- Nortriptyline (*Aventyl, Pamelor*) 10–100 mg qhs [T: 10, 25, 50, 75]; desipramine (*Norpramin*) 10–75 mg qam [T: 10, 25, 50, 75]
- Carbamazepine: (*Tegretol*) 200–400 mg tid [T: 100, 200; S: 100 mg/5 mL]; (*Tegretol XR*) 200 mg bid [T: 100, 200, 400]
- Gabapentin (*Neurontin*) 100–600 mg tid [C: 100, 300, 400; T: 600, 800]
- Capsaicin cream (eg, *Zostrix*) 0.075% applied tid–qid [0.025%, 0.075%]
- Transcutaneous electrical nerve stimulation may be of benefit.
- Lidocaine 5% patches (*Lidoderm*) 1–3 patches covering the affected area up to 12 h/d [700 mg patch] is useful for post-herpetic neuralgia.

Figure 4. Algorithm for Diagnosis of Peripheral Neuropathy

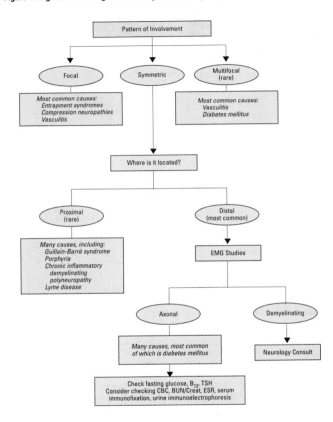

Source: Data from Poncelet AN. An algorithm for the evaluation of peripheral neuropathy. *Am Fam Phys.* 1998;57(4):755–764.

COMMONLY USED DEFINITIONS
- Established osteoporosis: occurrence of a minimal trauma fracture of any bone (WHO).
- Osteoporosis: a skeletal disorder characterized by compromised bone strength (bone density and bone quality) predisposing to an increased risk of fracture: NIH Consensus Development Panel. Osteoporosis prevention, diagnosis, and therapy. *JAMA* 2001; 285 (6):785–795.
- Osteoporosis: bone mineral density 2.5 SD or more below that of younger normal individuals (T score) (WHO).

RISK FACTORS FOR OSTEOPOROTIC FRACTURE
- Previous fracture as adult
- Dementia
- Depression
- Low calcium intake
- Low physical activity
- Fracture in 1st-degree relative
- Frailty
- Alcoholism
- Female sex
- Weight < 127 lb if female
- Cigarette smoking
- Early menopause
- Recurrent falls

TOXINS AND MEDICATIONS THAT CAN CAUSE OR AGGRAVATE OSTEOPOROSIS
- Alcohol (in excess)
- Anticonvulsants
- Corticosteroids
- Heparin
- Lithium
- Phenytoin
- Smoking
- Thyroxine (if overreplaced or in suppressive doses)

EVALUATION
Some experts recommend excluding secondary causes (serum PTH, TSH, calcium, phosphorus, albumin, alkaline phosphatase, bioavailable testosterone in men, renal and liver function tests, CBC, UA, electrolytes). Less consensus on: vitamin D levels, 24-h urinary calcium excretion; BMD test only if results could influence treatment.

MANAGEMENT
Universal Recommendations
- Calcium 1200 mg/d
- Vitamin D 400–800 IU
- Avoid tobacco
- Weight-bearing exercise
- Falls prevention
- No more than moderate alcohol use

Pharmacologic Prevention
- Women over 70 with multiple risk factors are at high enough risk to initiate treatment without BMD testing.
- Some organizations have recommended initiating pharmacologic management in women with BMD T scores below −2 in the absence of risk factors and in women with T scores below −1.5 if other risk factors are present.
- Regimens:
  - Estrogen (see **Table 81** for dosing) *or*

- Alendronate (*Fosamax*) 5 mg/d or 35 mg/wk [T: 5, 10, 35, 40, 70] (must be taken fasting with water; patient must remain upright and npo for at least 30 min after taking; relatively contraindicated in GERD) *or*
- Risedronate (*Actonel*) 5 mg/d [T: 5, 30] (must be taken fasting or at least 2 h after evening meal; patient must remain upright and npo for 30 min after taking) *or*
- Raloxifene (*Evista*) 60 mg/d [T: 60].

Pharmacologic Treatment
- Estrogen (see **Table 81** for dosing) *or*
- Alendronate (*Fosamax*) 10 mg/d or 70 mg/wk [T: 5, 10, 35, 40, 70] (must be taken fasting with water; patient must remain upright and npo for at least 30 min after taking; relatively contraindicated in GERD) *or*
- Risedronate (*Actonel*) 5 mg/d [T: 5, 30] (must be taken fasting or at least 2 h after evening meal; patient must remain upright and npo for 30 min after taking) *or*
- Raloxifene (*Evista*) 60 mg/d [T: 60] *or*
- Calcitonin (*Calcimar, Cibacalcin, Miacalcin, Osteocalcin, Salmonine*) 100 IU/d SC [Inj: human (*Cibacalcin*) 0.5 mg/vial; salmon 200 units/mL) or 200 IU (*Miacalcin*) [200 units/activation] (intranasally, alternate nostrils every other day). May also be helpful for analgesic effect in patients with acute vertebral fracture.

Table 59. Bone Outcomes, Level of Evidence,* and Cost of Drugs for Osteoporosis				
Drug	Spine BMD and Fracture	Hip BMD	Hip Fracture	All Nonspinal Fractures
Estrogen**	improved–R	improved–R	reduced–O	no effect–R
Raloxifene	improved–R	improved–R	no data	no effect–R
Alendronate	improved–R	improved–R	reduced–R	reduced–R
Risedronate	improved–R	improved–R	reduced–R	reduced–R
Calcitonin (nasal)	improved–R	no effect–R	no effect–R	no effect–R

* The populations studied, sample sizes of individual studies, and duration of follow-up vary considerably; hence, this summary must be interpreted cautiously. Moreover, several randomized clinical trials are currently in progress and new findings may appear.
** The least expensive of the drugs listed.
Note: O = observational study; R = randomized clinical trial.

Table 60. Effects on Other Outcomes, Level of Evidence,* and Risks of Drugs for Osteoporosis						
Drug	CHD Risk Factors	CHD Prevention	CHD Treatment	Breast Cancer	Deep-Vein Thrombosis	Other
Estrogen	improved–R	improved–O	no effect–R	↑ risk–O	↑ risk–R	↑ vaginal bleeding–R
Raloxifene	improved–R	no data	no data	↓ risk–R	↑ risk–R	↑ hot flushes–R
Alendronate	no data	no data	no data	no data	no data	esophagitis
Risedronate	no data	no data	no data	no data	no data	
Calcitonin (nasal)	no data	no data	no data	no data	no data	rhinitis in 10%–12%

* The populations studied, sample sizes of individual studies, and duration of follow-up vary considerably; hence, this summary must be interpreted cautiously. Moreover, several randomized clinical trials are currently in progress and new findings may appear.
Note: CHD = coronary heart disease; O = observational study; R = randomized clinical trial.

PAIN

DEFINITION
An unpleasant sensory and emotional experience associated with actual or potential tissue damage

Acute Pain
Distinct onset, obvious pathology, short duration; common causes: surgery (postoperatively), headache

Chronic Pain
Persistent > 3 mo, often associated with functional and psychologic impairment, can fluctuate in character and intensity over time; common causes: arthritis, cancer, claudication, leg cramps, neuropathy, radiculopathy

EVALUATION
Key Points, Approach
- Assume patient's report is the most reliable evidence of pain intensity.
- Assess for pain on each presentation (older adults may be reluctant to report pain).
- Use synonyms for pain (eg, burning, aching, soreness, discomfort).
- Use a standard pain scale (see p 170); adapt for sensory impairments (eg, large print, written versus spoken).
- Assess cognitively impaired patients by:
  - Using simple tools or questions with yes/no answers.
  - Noting increased vocalizations (eg, moaning, groaning, crying).
  - Observing behaviors (eg, grimacing, irritability, failure to move an extremity, guarding).
  - Asking caregiver about recent changes in function, gait, behavior patterns, mood.
- Reassess regularly for improvement, deterioration, complications; keep log.
- Refer for comprehensive multidisciplinary evaluation for complex pain problem.

History and Physical
- Focus on a complete examination of pain source.
- Distinguish new illness from chronic condition.
- Analgesic history: effectiveness and side effects, current and previous prescription drugs, OTC drugs, "natural" remedies.
- Lab and diagnostic tests: to establish etiologic diagnosis.

Present Pain Complaint
Provocative (aggravating) and **P**alliative (relieving) factors
Quality (eg, burning, stabbing, dull, throbbing)
Region
Severity (eg, scale of 0 for no pain to 10 for worst pain possible; see p 171)
Timing (eg, when pain occurs, frequency and duration)

Psychosocial Assessment
Depression (see p 165 for screen), anxiety, mental status (see p 161 for screen).

Functional Assessment
ADLs, impact on activities (see pp 163–164 for screens) and quality of life.

Brief Pain Inventory
Use for comprehensive assessment of pain and its impact. See, eg, the short form in Management of Cancer Pain Guidelines Panel. *Management of Cancer Pain.* Clinical Practice Guidelines No. 9. Rockville, MD: AHCPR, Public Health Service, US Dept of Health and Human Services; March 1994. AHCPR Publication No. 94-0592.

PAIN MANAGEMENT
Acute Pain and Short-Term Management
• For severe pain, consider patient-controlled analgesic pump.
• Use fixed schedule of acetaminophen or opioids.
• Include nonpharmacologic strategies (eg, relaxation, heat or cold).

Chronic Pain
• Use multidisciplinary assessment and treatment.
• Educate patient for self-management and coping.
• Combine drug and nondrug strategies.
• Anticipate and attend to depression and anxiety.

Nonpharmacologic Treatment
• Educate patient and caregiver.
• Emphasize self-administered therapies (eg, heat, cold, massage, liniments and topical agents).
• Prescribe exercise, especially for chronic pain.
• Add therapy conducted by professionals (eg, distraction, relaxation techniques, music therapy, coping skills, biofeedback, imagery, hypnosis) as needed.
• When appropriate, obtain:
  - Rehabilitation medicine consult (OT, PT) for mechanical devices to minimize pain and facilitate activity (eg, splints), transcutaneous electrical nerve stimulation, range-of-motion and ADL programs.
  - Psychiatric pain management consult for somatization or hysteria, management of withdrawal.
  - Anesthesia pain consult for nerve blocks, neuroablation for neuropathic conditions not relieved by other treatments (eg, post-herpetic neuralgia, lumbar spinal stenosis, neuropathy).

Pharmacologic Treatment
Selection of Agent(s):
• Base initial choice of analgesic on the severity and type of pain:
  - Consider nonopioids for mild pain (rating 0–3) (see **Table 51**).
  - Consider weak opioids (see **Table 61**), often in combination with a nonopioid, for mild to moderate pain (rating 4–6) (eg, codeine, oxycodone, hydrocodone, tramadol).
  - Consider strong opioids for more severe pain (rating 7–10) (eg, morphine, hydromorphone, oxymorphone).

- Consider adjuvant drugs (see **Table 62**) alone or in conjunction with opioids or nonopioids for neuropathic pain and other selected chronic conditions.
- Select lowest side-effect profile agents.
- Select least invasive route (usually oral) and fast-onset, short-acting analgesics for episodic or breakthrough pain.
- Use long-acting or sustained-release analgesics for continuous pain.
- Use NSAIDs with caution (avoid if abnormal renal function, hx of peptic ulcer disease, bleeding diathesis) (see **Table 51**).
- Consider COX-2 inhibitors for patients who would benefit from anti-inflammatory drug therapy but who are at high risk for NSAID-induced peptic ulcer disease.
- Consider fixed-dose combinations (eg, acetaminophen and codeine) for mild to moderate pain; do not exceed maximum dose for nonopioid or NSAID.
- Avoid using multiple opioids or nonopioids when possible.
- Use drugs with long half-life with caution (eg, methadone or levorphanol, fentanyl patch, particularly in opioid-naive patients); titrate slowly; effective activity may exceed stated duration.

Adjustment of Dosage:
- Begin with lowest dose possible, increasing slowly.
- Titrate dose on basis of persistent need for and use of medications for breakthrough pain. If using 3 or more doses of breakthrough pain medication per day, increase dose of sustained-release medication.
- Dose to therapeutic ceiling of nonopioid or NSAID if side effects permit.
- Increase opioid dose until pain relief achieved or side effects unmanageable before changing drugs (there is no maximum dose or analgesic ceiling with opioids).
- Use morphine equivalents as a common denominator for all dose conversion to avoid errors.
- When changing opioids, decrease equianalgesic dose by 50% because of incomplete crossover.
- Administer around-the-clock for continuous pain.
- Reassess, re-examine, and readjust therapy frequently until pain is relieved.

Management of Side Effects:
- Anticipate, prevent, and vigorously treat side effects; expect older patients to be more sensitive to side effects.
- Begin prophylactic laxative, osmotic, or stimulant when initiating opioid therapy (see **Table 34**); if patient taking sufficient fluids, increase fiber or psyllium; titrate laxative dose up with opiate dose.
- Monitor for sedation, delirium, urinary retention, constipation, respiratory depression, and nausea; tolerance develops to mild sedation, nausea, and impaired cognitive function.
- On long-term NSAID use, monitor periodically for GI blood loss, renal insufficiency, and other drug-drug and drug-disease interactions.
- Use the following drugs only with extreme caution: carisoprodol, chlorzoxazone, cyclobenzaprine, indomethacin, meperidine, metaxalone, methocarbamol, nalbuphine, pentazocine, propoxyphene (see also p 178 for HCFA criteria regarding inappropriate drug use).

Table 61. Opioid Analgesic Drugs				
Class, Drug	**MS Equiv* (Route)**	**Starting Oral Dosage**	**Formulations**	**Indication for Pain****
Short-acting Drugs				
Codeine	200 mg (po)	30–60 mg q 4–6 h	[T: 15, 30, 60; Inj: 30, 60]	A
Codeine & acetaminophen†	NA	1–2 tabs q 4–6 h; if 1 tab used, add 325 mg acetaminophen	[T: 15/325, 30/325, 60/325, 30/500, 30/650, 7.5/300, 15/300, 30/300, 60/300; S: 12/120/5mL]	A
Hydrocodone & acetaminophen† (eg, *Lorcet, Lortab, Vicodin*)	ND	5–10 mg q 4–6 h	[T: 10/325, 5/400, 7.5/400, 10/400, 2.5/500, 5/500, 7.5/500, 10/500, 7.5/650, 7.5/750, 10/650, 10/660; C: 5/500; S: 2.5/167/5 mL (contains 7% alcohol)]	A
& aspirin (eg, *Lortab ASA*)			[T: 5/500]	
& ibuprofen (eg, *Vicoprofen*)			[T: 7.5/200]	
Oxycodone (*Oxy IR, Roxicodone*)	20 mg (po)	5–10 mg q 3–4 h	[T: 5; C: 5; S: 5 mg/mL, 20 mg/mL]	A
(*Percocet, Tylox* with acetaminophen†)			[T: 5/325; C: 5/500; S: 5/325/5 mL]	
(*Percodan* with aspirin)			[T: 2.44/325, 4.88/325]	
Morphine (*MSIR, Astramorph PF, Duramorph, Infumorph, Roxanol, OMS Concentrate, MS/L, RMS, MS/S*)	30 mg (po), 10 mg (IV)	10–30 mg q 4–6 h	[T: 15, 30; soluble T: 10, 15, 30; Inj: 0.5, 1–5, 8, 10, 15, 25, 50 mg/mL; S: 10, 20, 100 mg/5 mL, 4, 20 mg/mL; Sp: 5, 10, 20, 30; plus injection solutions]	B
Hydromorphone (*Dilaudid, Hydrostat*)	7.5 mg (po), 1.5 mg (IV), 6 mg (rectal)	1–2 mg q 3–4 h	[T: 1, 2, 3, 4, 8; S: 5 mg/5 mL; Inj: 1–4, 10 mg/mL; Sp: 3]	B
Oxymorphone (*Numorphan*)	1 mg (IV), 10 mg (rectal)	5 mg q 4–6 h	[Inj: 1, 1.5 mg/mL; Sp: 5]	B
Fentanyl (*Actiq, Fentanyl Oralet*)	NA	2.5–5 mg/kg; suck on lozenges, effect begins within 10 min	[T: 200, 300, 400, 600, 800, 1200, 1600 µg]	B

Table 61. Opioid Analgesic Drugs (cont.)				
Class, Drug	MS Equiv* (Route)	Starting Oral Dosage	Formulations	Indication for Pain**
Tramadol (*Ultram*)	NA	50–100 mg q 4–6 h	[T: 50, 100, 150, 300]	B
Long-acting Drugs				
SR morphine (*MS Contin, Kadian, Oramorph SR*)	30 mg	15–30 mg q 8–12 h or 24 h equiv of total prior analgesics in divided doses q 12 h	[CR: 15, 30, 60, 100, 200]	B
SR oxycodone (*OxyContin*)	20–30 mg	10–20 mg q 12 h or 24 h equiv of total prior analgesics in divided doses q 12 h	[CR: 10, 20, 40, 80, 160]	B
Transdermal fentanyl (*Duragesic*)	NA (see package insert)	25 mg/h or higher	[25 µg/h (10 cm²), 50 µg/h (20 cm²), 75 µg/h (30 cm²), 100 µg/h (40 cm²)]	B

* MS Equiv = morphine sulfate equivalent dose; morphine equivalency = dose of opioid equivalent to 10 mg of oral morphine or 30 mg of parenteral morphine. NA = not applicable; ND = no data available.
** A = mild to moderate pain; B = moderate to severe pain.
† Caution: total acetaminophen dose should not exceed 4 g/d.
Note: All are metabolized by liver and excreted primarily in urine. Renal or hepatic dysfunction may cause prolonged duration and cumulative effects.

Table 62. Adjuvant Drugs for Pain Relief in Elderly Patients			
Class, Drug	Formulations	Starting Dosage	Comments
Antiarrhythmics Mexiletine (*Mexitil*)	[C: 150, 200, 250]	150 mg bid–qid	Side effects such as tremor, dizziness, unsteadiness, paresthesias are common; rarely, hepatic damage and blood dyscrasias occur; avoid use in patients with preexisting heart disease; start with low dose and titrate slowly; recommend initial and follow-up ECGs; titrate to tid–qid dosing
Anticonvulsants (see **Table 57**)			If one does not work, try another
Antidepressants (see **Table 23**)			Use low-dose desipramine or nortriptyline; data on SSRIs lacking
Corticosteroids (see **Table 27**)			Low-dose medical management may be helpful in inflammatory conditions

(continues)

Table 62. Adjuvant Drugs for Pain Relief in Elderly Patients (cont.)

Class, Drug	Formulations	Starting Dosage	Comments
Counterirritants Camphor-menthol-phenol (*Sarna*)*	[lotion: camphor 5%, menthol 5%, phenol 5%]	prn	May be effective for arthritic pain, but effect limited when pain affects multiple joints; can cause skin injury, especially if used with heat or occlusive dressing
Camphor & phenol (*Campho-Phenique*)*	[liquid: camphor 5%, phenol 4.7%]	prn	
Methylsalicylate and menthol			
(*Ben-Gay* ointment,* *Icy Hot* cream*)	[methylsalicylate 18.3%, menthol 16%]	3–4 × / d	Apply to affected area
(*Ben-Gay* extra strength cream*)	[methylsalicylate 30%, menthol 10%]	3–4 × / d	Apply to affected area
Trolamine salicylate (*Aspercreme* rub*)	[trolamine salicylate 10%]	≤ 4 × / d	Apply to affected area
Other agents			
Baclofen (*Lioresal*)	[10, 20; Inj. 500 µg/mL, 2000 µg/mL]	5 mg bid–tid	Probably increased sensitivity and decreased clearance; monitor for weakness, urinary dysfunction; avoid abrupt discontinuation because of CNS irritability
Capsaicin (eg, *Capsin*, *Capzasin*, *No Pain-HP*, *R-Gel, Zostrix*)	[creams, lotions, gels, roll-on: 0.025%, 0.075%]	3–4 × / d	Renders skin and joints insensitive by depleting and preventing reaccumulation of substance P in peripheral sensory neurons; may cause burning sensation; instruct patient to wash hands after application to prevent eye contact; do not apply to open or broken skin

* Available over-the-counter.
Note: Various adjuvant classes are useful for the treatment of neuropathic pain. Tricyclic antidepressants are often helpful for migraine or tension headaches and arthritic conditions. Baclofen is particularly useful for muscle-related problems, such as spasms.

PALLIATIVE AND END-OF-LIFE CARE

DEFINITION
"The active total care of patients, controlling pain and minimizing emotional, social and spiritual problems at a time when disease is not responsive to active treatment" (WHO, 1990).

PRINCIPLES
- Support, educate, and treat both patient and family.
- Address physical, psychologic, social, and spiritual needs.
- Use multidisciplinary team (physicians, nurses, social workers, chaplain, pharmacist, physical and occupational therapists, dietitian, family and caregivers, volunteers).
- Focus on symptom management.
- Make care available 24 h/d, 7 d/wk.
- Offer bereavement support.
- Supply therapeutic environment (palliation can be given in any location).
- Provide for all dying patients.

QUALITY OF LIFE
Ways to help patient and family enhance quality of life at the end of life:
- Communicate, listen
- Teach stress management, coping
- Use all available resources
- Support decision making
- Encourage conflict resolution
- Help complete unfinished business
- Urge focus on non-illness-related affairs
- Urge a focus on one day at a time
- Help anticipate grief, losses
- Help focus on attainable goals
- Encourage spiritual practices
- Promote physical, psychologic comfort

END-OF-LIFE DECISIONS
Follow principles involved in informed decision making (see **Figure 2**).

Hospice Referral
- Patients, families, or other health care provides can refer, but a physician's order is required for admission to a hospice program.
- Referral is appropriate when aggressive, curative treatment is stopped. Physician's certification of life expectancy < 6 mo required for Medicare hospice benefit.
- Hospice must be accepted by the patient or family, or both, and can be rescinded at any time.
- Hospice provides medications (not routine), equipment, team member visits, home health aides, and volunteers.
- Optimal hospice care requires adequate time in the program; referral when death is imminent does not take full advantage of hospice care.

Advance Directives
Designed to respect patient's autonomy and determine his/her wishes about future life-sustaining medical treatment if unable to indicate wishes.

Oral Statements
- Conversations with relatives, friends, clinicians are most common form; should be thoroughly documented in medical record for later reference.
- Properly verified oral statements carry same ethical and legal weight as those recorded in writing.

Instructional Advance Directives (DNR Orders, Living Wills)
- Written instructions regarding the initiation, continuation, withholding, or withdrawal of particular forms of life-sustaining medical treatment.
- May be revoked or altered at any time by the patient.
- Clinicians who comply with such directives are provided legal immunity for such actions.

Durable Power of Attorney for Health Care or Health Care Proxy
A written document that enables a capable person to appoint someone else to make future medical treatment choices for him or her in the event of decisional incapacity.

Key Interventions, Treatment Decisions to Include in Advance Directives:
- Resuscitation procedures
- Mechanical respiration
- Chemotherapy, radiation therapy
- Dialysis
- Simple diagnostic tests
- Pain control
- Blood products, transfusions
- Terminal sedation

Withholding or Withdrawing Therapy
- There is no ethical or legal difference between withholding an intervention (not starting it) and withdrawing life-sustaining medical treatment (stopping it after it has been started).
- Beginning a treatment does not preclude stopping it later; a time-limited trial may be appropriate.
- Palliative care should not be limited, even if life-sustaining treatments are withdrawn or withheld.
- Decisions on artificial feeding should be based on the same criteria applied to ventilators and other medical treatment.

Euthanasia
- Active euthanasia: direct intervention, such as lethal injection, intended to hasten a patient's death; a criminal act of homicide.
- Passive euthanasia: withdrawal or withholding of unwanted or unduly burdensome life-sustaining treatment; appropriate in certain circumstances.
- Assisted suicide: the patient's intentional, willful ending of his/her own life with the assistance of another; a criminal offense in most states.

MANAGEMENT OF COMMON END-OF-LIFE SYMPTOMS
Pain
- The most distressing symptom for patients and caregivers.
- If intent is to relieve suffering, the risk that sufficient medication will produce an unintended effect (hastening death) is morally acceptable.
- Primary goal: to alleviate suffering at end of life. See Pain (p 107) for assessment and interventions.

- Alternate routes may be needed, eg, transdermal, transmucosal, rectal, vaginal, topical, epidural, and intrathecal.
- Recommend expert pain management consult if pain not adequately relieved with standard analgesic guidelines and interventions.
- Additional treatment may include:
  - radionuclides and bisphosphonates (for metastatic bone pain).
  - treatments (eg, radiotherapy, chemotherapy) directed at source of pain.
- Pain crisis: Sedation at end of life for intractable pain and suffering is an important option to discuss with patients. Ketamine (*Ketalar*) 0.1 mg/kg IV bolus. Repeat as needed q 5 min. Follow with infusion of 0.015 mg/kg/min IV (SC if IV access not available at 0.3–0.5 mg/kg). Decrease opioid dose by 50%. Benzodiazepine may be useful. Observe for problems with increased secretions and treat (see section on excessive secretions).

Weakness, Fatigue
Nonpharmacologic:
- Modify environment to decrease energy expenditure (eg, placement of phone, bedside commode, and drinks).
- Adjust room temperature to patient's comfort.
- Teach energy-conserving techniques (eg, reordering tasks—eating first, resting, then bathing).
- Modify daily procedures (eg, sitting while showering, not standing).
Pharmacologic:
- Treat remediable causes such as pain, medication toxicity, insomnia, anemia, and depression.
- Consider psychostimulants (eg, dextroamphetamine [*Dexedrine*] 2.5 mg po qam or bid *or* methylphenidate [*Ritalin*] 5–10 mg po qam or bid); monitor for signs of psychosis, agitation, or sleep disturbance.

Dysphagia
Nonpharmacologic:
- Feed small, frequent amounts of pureed or soft foods.
- Avoid spicy, salty, acidic, sticky, and extremely hot or cold foods.
- Keep head of bed elevated for 30 min after eating.
- Instruct patient to wear dentures and to chew thoroughly.
- Use suction machine when necessary.
Pharmacologic:
- For painful mucositis: 1:2:8 mixture of diphenhydramine elixir: lidocaine [2%–4%]: *Maalox* as a swish-and-swallow suspension before meals.
- For candidiasis: clotrimazole 10 mg troches, 5 doses/d, *or* fluconazole 150 mg po followed by 100 mg po qd × 5 d.
- For severe halitosis: antimicrobial mouthwash; metronidazole 250–500 mg po tid or applied as a topical gel [0.75%], if feasible.

Dyspnea
Nonpharmacologic:
- Teach positions to facilitate breathing, elevate head of bed.
- Teach relaxation techniques.
- Eliminate smoke and allergens.
- Administer oxygen.

Pharmacologic:
- Opioids: oral morphine concentrate (20 mg/mL): 1/4 to 1/2 mL sl/po; repeat in 10–15 min prn); nebulized morphine 2.5 mg in 2–4 cc NS or fentanyl 25–50 µg in 2–4 cc NS; or IV morphine 1 mg or equivalent opioid q 5–10 min.
- Bronchodilators (see **Table 73**).
- Diuretics, if evidence of volume overload (see **Table 16**).
- Anxiolytics (eg, lorazepam po/sl/SC 0.5–2 mg q 2–4 h or prn); titrate slowly to effect.

Constipation
Most common cause: side effects of opioids, medications with anticholinergic side-effects (see **Table 34**).

Bowel Obstruction
Indications for Radiographic Evaluation:
- To differentiate constipation and mechanical obstruction
- To confirm the obstruction, determine site and nature if surgery is being considered

Nonpharmacologic Management:
- Nasogastric intubation: only if surgery is being considered, for high-level obstructions, and poor response to pharmacotherapy
- Percutaneous venting gastrostomy: for high-level obstructions and profuse vomiting not responsive to antiemetics
- Palliative surgery
- Hydration: IV or hypodermoclysis

Pharmacologic Management (aimed at specific symptoms):
- Nausea and vomiting: haloperidol (*Haldol*) po, IM 0.5–5 mg (≤ 10 mg) q 4–8 h prn; ondansetron (*Zofran*) IV (over 2–5 min) 4 mg q 12 h, po 8 mg q 12 h (L) [Inj; T: 4, 8]; see also **Table 35**.
- Spasm, pain, and vomiting: scopolamine IM, IV, SC 0.3–0.65 mg q 4–6 h prn; oral 0.4–0.8 mg q 4–8 h prn; transdermal 2.5 cm² patch applied behind the ear q 3 d (L) [Inj; T: 0.4; patch 1.5 mg] or hyoscyamine (*Levsin/SL*) sublingual [T: 0.125; S: 0.125 mg/mL] 0.125–0.25 tid–qid.
- Diarrhea and excessive secretions: loperamide (*Imodium A-D*) see **Table 36**; octreotide (*Sandostatin*) SC 0.15–0.3 mg q 12 h (L) [Inj], very expensive.
- Pain: see **Table 61**.
- Inflammation due to malignant obstruction: dexamethasone (*Decadron*) oral: 4 mg qid × 5–7 d.

Excessive Secretions
Non pharmacologic: Positioning and suctioning, as needed
Pharmacologic: Glycopyrrolate 0.1–0.4 mg IV/SC q 4 h prn or scopolomine 0.3–0.6 mg SC prn or transdermal scopolomine patch q 72 h or atropine 0.3–0.5 mg SC, sublingual, nebulized q 4 h prn

Cough See Respiratory Diseases (p 135).

Nausea, Vomiting See Gastrointestinal Diseases (p 59).

Malnutrition, Dehydration See also Malnutrition (p 84).
Nonpharmacologic:
- Educate patient and family on effects of disease progression resulting in lack of appetite and weight loss.
- Promote interest, enjoyment in meals (eg, alcoholic beverage if desired, involve patient in meal planning, small frequent feedings, cold or semi-frozen nutritional drinks).
- Good oral care is important.

Pharmacologic:
- Corticosteroids: Dexamethasone 1–2 mg po tid; methylprednisolone 1–2 mg po bid; prednisone 5 mg po tid.
- Hormone therapy: Megestrol acetate 200–800 mg qd.

Altered Mental Status, Delirium See Delirium (p 35).

Anxiety, Depression
- Provide opportunity to discuss feelings, fears, existential concerns
- Referral to appropriate team members (spiritual, nursing)
- Medicate (see Anxiety, p 17, and Depression, p 42).

Source: Fine P. *Hospice Companion—Processes to Optimize Care During the Last Phase of Life.* Scottsdale, AZ: VistaCare, Inc.; 1998.

117

PREOPERATIVE CARE
Cardiac Risk Assessment
Assess patient for risk of perioperative cardiac complications (MI, pulmonary edema, cardiac arrest):
1. Collect variables from the Modified Cardiac Risk Index (see **Table 63**).
2. If surgery is emergent, proceed directly to surgery.
3. If surgery is nonemergent, apply algorithm in **Figure 5**.

Table 63. Modified Cardiac Risk Index (see step 1, above, and Figure 5)	
Variable	**Points**
Coronary artery disease	
MI < 6 months earlier	10
MI > 6 months earlier	5
Canadian Cardiovascular Society angina classification*	
Class III	10
Class IV	20
Alveolar pulmonary edema	
Within 1 wk	10
Ever	5
Suspected critical aortic stenosis	20
Arrhythmias	
Rhythm other than sinus or sinus plus atrial premature beats on ECG	5
> 5 premature ventricular contractions on ECG	5
Poor general medical status, defined as any of the following: $Po_2 < 60$ mm Hg, $Pco_2 > 50$ mm Hg, K^+ level < 3.0 mg/dL, BUN level > 50 mg/dL (18 mmol/L), creatinine level > 3 mg/dL (260 mmol/L), bedridden	5
Age > 70 years	5
Emergency surgery	10

*Class III = angina with walking one to two level blocks or climbing one flight of stairs or less at a normal pace; Class IV = inability to perform any physical activity without development of angina.
Source: Detsky AS, Abrams HO, McLaughlin JR, et al. Predicting cardiac complications in patients undergoing non-cardiac surgery. *J Gen Intern Med.* 1986;1:211–219. Reprinted by permission of Blackwell Science, Inc.

Pulmonary Risk Assessment
Assessing the patient for risk of pulmonary complications (respiratory failure, pneumonia, atelectasis) includes the following risk factors:
Smoking: To lower risk, patients should quit at least 8 wk prior to surgery.
COPD: Bronchodilators, physical therapy, antibiotics, and corticosteroids given preoperatively can reduce risk.
ASA Class: III—severe systemic disease; IV—life-threatening systemic disease; V—moribund.
Surgical Site: Upper abdominal, thoracic, > 3-h surgeries pose the greatest increased risk.

Note: Routine spirometry has not been shown to be useful in risk assessment.

Figure 5. Coronary Risk Assessment of Nonemergent, Noncardiac Surgery

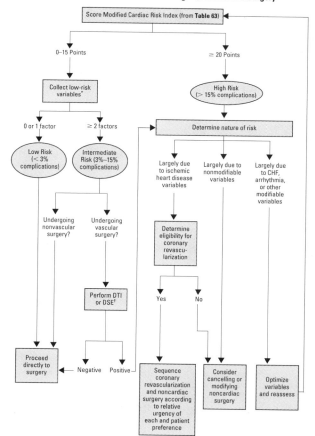

*Low-risk variables = age > 70 yr, hx of angina, diabetes mellitus, Q waves on ECG, hx of MI, ST-segment ischemic abnormalities on resting ECG, hypertension with severe LVH, hx of CHF.

†DTI = dipyridamole thallium imaging; DSE = dobutamine stress echocardiogram.

Source: Adapted from: Appendix Figure 1 from American College of Physicians. Clinical guideline, part 1: guidelines for assessing and managing perioperative risk from coronary artery disease associated with major noncardiac surgery. *Ann Intern Med.* 1997;127:309–312. Reprinted with permission.

Other Assessments

Cognitive Status: Unrecognized dementia is a risk factor for postoperative delirium. Measure preoperative cognitive status with Mini-Cog (see p 161) or MMSE.

Nutritional Status: Poor nutritional status can impair wound healing. Measure height, weight, serum albumin.

Routine Laboratory Tests: Recommended: Hemoglobin and hematocrit, electrolytes, creatinine, BUN, ECG, CXR, albumin. Optional: CBC, platelets, ABG, PT, PTT.

Cataract Surgery: Routine laboratory testing or cardiopulmonary risk assessment is unneccessary for cataract surgery performed under local anesthesia.

Advance Directives: Establish or update.

PERIOPERATIVE MANAGEMENT

β-Blocker Use

Patients with diagnosed CAD or with > 2 risk factors for CAD (male gender, hypertension, smoking, diabetes mellitus, dyslipidemia, obesity, family history, sedentary life style) should receive perioperative atenolol (*Tenormin*), unless heart rate is < 55 beats/min; SBP < 100; or the patient has asthma, CHF, or third-degree heart block. Give two doses of atenolol IV, 5 mg administered over 5 min, the first 30 min before surgery, the second immediately after surgery. Following surgery, begin atenolol 50–100 mg po qd until discharge.

Endocarditis Prophylaxis

Depends on cardiac condition and type of procedure (see pp 125–127).

DVT Prophylaxis (see also pp 14–16)

General Surgery: Elastic stockings plus LDUH, 5000 units SC 2 h before surgery and q 12 h after surgery; for higher risk, consider LDUH q 8 h, LMWH (enoxaparin [*Lovenox*] 30 mg SC q 12 h), and/or the use of IPC devices

Total Hip Replacement: LMWH, low-molecular-weight heparinoid (danaparoid [*Orgaran*] 750 anti-Xa units SC q 12 h), or warfarin (adjust INR 2.0 to 3.0) or dose-adjusted heparin

Total Knee Replacement: LMWH or IPC

Surgical Hip Fracture Repair: IPC plus either LMWH or warfarin

Common Problems to Monitor

- Confusion: see p 35
- Intra- and postoperative coronary events: postoperative ECG to check
- Malnutrition: see p 84
- Pain: see p 107
- Polypharmacy: review medications daily
- Pulmonary complications: minimized by incentive spirometry, coughing, early ambulation
- Rehabilitation: encourage early mobility
- Skin breakdown: see p 121

PRESSURE ULCERS

DEFINITION
Any lesion caused by unrelieved pressure resulting in damage of underlying tissue; usually occurs over bony prominence.

EXTRINSIC RISK FACTORS
- Pressure
- Shear
- Friction

INTRINSIC RISK FACTORS
- Immobility (eg, chairbound)
- ↑ Age
- Malnutrition
- Moisture (eg, incontinence)
- Diabetes mellitus
- Stroke
- ↓ Blood pressure
- ↑ Body temperature
- White race

EVALUATION
- Screen for presence of intrinsic risk factors (see above).
- Determine intensity of risk status using validated tool, eg, Braden Scale; see Braden BJ, Bergstrom N. Clinical utility of the Braden Scale for predicting pressure sore risk. *Decubitus* 1989;2(3):44–51; for online versions of the scale:
  http://www.skinwound.com/online_training_manual/braden_scale.htm (for a downloadable PDF file)
  http://text.nlm.nih.gov (in AHCPR pressure ulcer practice guideline).
- Assess skin daily, especially persons with one or more risk factors.
- Determine severity of lesion by using staging criteria:
  - **Stage I:** An observable pressure-related alteration of intact skin whose indicators as compared with an adjacent or opposite area on the body may include changes in one or more of the following: skin temperature (warmth or coolness), tissue consistency (firm or boggy feel), and/or sensation (pain, itching). The ulcer appears as a defined area of persistent redness in lightly pigmented skin, whereas in darker skin tones, it may appear with persistent red, blue, or purple hues.
  - **Stage II:** Partial-thickness skin loss involving epidermis and/or dermis; presents as abrasion, blister, or shallow crater.
  - **Stage III:** Full-thickness skin loss involving damage or necrosis of subcutaneous tissue which may extend down to, but not through, underlying fascia; presents as deep crater with or without undermining of adjacent tissue.
  - **Stage IV:** Full-thickness skin loss with extensive destruction, tissue necrosis, or damage to muscle, bone, or supporting structures. May have associated undermining of sinus tracts. Note: eschar-covered ulcers cannot be staged until eschar is removed.
- No improvement over 2 wk should result in complete reassessment of risk factors and management strategies.
- Heel ulcers: Without signs of infection or inflammation, do not debride dry eschar. With signs of infection or inflammation or wet eschar, surgically debride; obtain vascular consult.

PREVENTION AND MANAGEMENT
Protect Wound and Surrounding Skin from Further Trauma
- Employ pressure-reduction strategies:
  - Reposition every 1–2 h.
  - Use pressure-reducing or relieving cushions, mattresses, and heel protectors.
  - Avoid doughnut cushions.
- Reduce friction and shear:
  - Maintain head of bed elevation < 30 degrees.
  - Use lift sheet.

Promote Clean Wound Bed, Prevent Infection
- Debride necrotic tissue, eschar:
  - Sharp: scissors, forceps, scalpel
  - Mechanical: wet-to-dry dressings
  - Autolytic: moisture-retentive dressings or hydrogels
  - Chemical: topical enzymes (eg, *Accuzyme, Santyl*)

Autolytic methods or topical enzymes may be used in conjunction with sharp debridement to facilitate more rapid removal of necrotic tissue.
- Cleansing:
  - Cleanse with each dressing change and as needed.
  - Use normal saline.
  - Irrigate using 8 mm Hg pressure (19-gauge IV catheter and 35-cc syringe) when wound is deep, tunneled, or undermined.

Maintain Moist Wound Environment
- Use moisture-retentive dressings:
  - Calcium alginate
  - Continuous moist saline gauze
  - Foams
  - Hydrogel
  - Hydrocolloids
  - Transparent films

Eliminate Dead Space
- Pack dead space (tunnels, undermining):
  - Moistened saline gauze dressings or strips
  - Calcium alginate dressings

Control Exudate
- Use exudate-absorbing dressings:
  - Calcium alginate dressings
  - Foam dressings
  - Moistened saline gauze dressings

Diagnose and Treat Infection
- Signs of infection:
  - Nonhealing wound despite optimal treatment
  - Foul odor to exudate
  - Friable granulation tissue
  - Wound breakdown
  - Increasing pain
  - Edema
  - Serous exudate with concurrent inflammation
  - Peri-wound heat, erythema

Swab culture is of limited value in diagnosing infection due to contaminated wound bed.
- Treatment of infection:
  - Remove necrotic tissue and purulent exudate from wound.
  - Use systemic antibiotics only in presence of spreading cellulitis, sepsis, or osteomyelitis.

Consider 2-wk trial of topical antibiotic for clean ulcers that are not healing or are continuing to produce exudate after 2–4 wk optimal care; antibiotic should be effective against gram-negative, gram-positive, and anaerobic organisms.

Support Healing Systemically
- Provide nutritional support (see p 84):
  - Increase calories and protein, including nutritional supplements as needed.
  - Obtain nutritional consult.
  - Use vitamin and mineral supplements.
- Provide adequate hydration with oral or parenteral fluids.

Surgical Repair
- Candidates: Stage IV pressure ulcers; severely undermined or tunneled wounds; ability to tolerate surgical procedure

Topical Wound Products

Table 64. Wound and Pressure Ulcer Products, by Drainage and Stage							
	Drainage			Wound Stage			
Product	Light	Moderate	Heavy	I	II	III	IV
Transparent film	X			X			
Foam island	X	X			X	X	
Hydrocolloids	X	X			X	X	
Petroleum-based nonadherent	X				X	X	
Alginate		X	X			X	X
Hydrogel	X				X	X	X
Gauze packing (moistened with saline)		X	X			X	X

Table 65. Common Dressings for Pressure Ulcer Treatment			
Dressing	Indications	Contraindications	Examples
Transparent film	Stage I ulcer Protection from friction Superficial scrape Autolytic debridement of slough Apply skin prep to intact skin to protect from adhesive	Skin tears Draining ulcers Suspicion of skin infection or fungus	*Bioclusive* *Tegaderm* *Op-site*
Foam island	Stage II, III Low to moderate exudate Can apply as window to secure transparent film	Excessive exudate Dry, crusted wound	*Alleyn* *Lyofoam*

(*continues*)
123

Table 65. Common Dressings for Pressure Ulcer Treatment (cont.)

Dressing	Indications	Contraindications	Examples
Hydrocolloids	Stage II, III Low to moderate drainage Good peri-wound skin integrity Autolytic debridement of slough Left in place 3–5 d Can apply as window to secure transparent film Can apply over alginate to control drainage Must control maceration Apply skin prep to intact skin to protect from adhesive	Poor skin integrity Infected ulcers Wound needs packing	*DuoDerm* *Extra thin film* *DuoDerm* *Tegasorb* *Replicare*
Petroleum-based nonadherent	Stage II, III Graft sites		*Vaseline gauze* *Xerofoam* *Adaptic*
Alginate	Stage II, III, IV Excessive drainage Apply dressing within wound borders Requires secondary dressing Must use skin prep Must control for maceration	Dry or minimally draining wound Superficial wounds with maceration	*Sorbsan* *Kaltostat* *Algosteril* *Algiderm*
Hydrogel (amorphous gels)	Stage II, III, IV Needs to be combined with gauze dressing Stays moist longer than saline gauze Changed 1–2 times/d Used as alternative to saline gauze for packing deep wounds with tunnels, undermining Reduces adherence of gauze to wound Must control for maceration	Macerated areas Wounds with excess exudate	*IntraSite gel* *Solosite gel*
(gel sheet)	Stage II Skin tears Needs to be held in place with topper dressing	Macerated areas Wounds with moderate to heavy exudate	*Vigilon*
Gauze packing	Stage III, IV Wounds with depth, especially those with tunnels, undermining		Square 2 × 2s, 4 × 4s *Fluffed Kerlix* *Plain Nugauze*
(moistened with saline)	Must be remoistened often to maintain moist wound environment		

Source: Copyright © 1999 by Rita Frantz. Used with permission.

PREVENTION

PREVENTIVE TESTS AND PROCEDURES

Table 66. Recommended Primary and Secondary Disease Prevention for Persons Aged 65 and Over

Preventive Strategy	Frequency
USPSTF* Recommendations for Primary Prevention	
BP screening	yearly
Influenza immunization	yearly
Obesity (height and weight)	yearly
Pneumonia immunization	once at age 65**
Smoking cessation	at every office visit
Tetanus immunization	every 10 yr
USPSTF* Recommendations for Secondary Prevention	
FOBT and/or sigmoidoscopy	yearly/every 3–5 yr
Hearing impairment screening	yearly
Mammography, clinical breast examination***	every 1–2 yr
Pap smear†	at least every 3 yr
Visual impairment screening	yearly
Other‡ Recommendations for Primary Prevention	
Aspirin to prevent MI	daily
Cholesterol screening	every 5 yr
Diabetes mellitus screening	yearly
HRT (see p 159)	daily
Other‡ Recommendations for Secondary Prevention	
Skin examination	yearly
Breast self-examination	monthly
Bone densitometry	(see p 105)
Cognitive impairment screening	yearly
PSA and digital rectal examination	yearly
TSH in women	yearly

*US Preventive Services Task Force. *Guide to Clinical Preventive Services.* 2nd ed. Baltimore: Williams and Wilkins; 1996. Or see: http://odphp.osophs.dhhs.gov/pubs/guidecps/
**Consider repeating pneumococcal vaccine every 6–7 yr.
***Mammograms to age 70 are virtually universally recommended; many organizations, including the USPSTF, recommend that mammography should be continued in women over 70 who have a reasonable life expectancy.
† Pap smear testing can be stopped at age 65. See p 158.
‡ Not endorsed by USPSTF for all older adults, but recommended in selected patients or by other professional organizations.

ENDOCARDITIS PROPHYLAXIS (AHA GUIDELINES)
Antibiotic Regimens Recommended (see Table 67)

Cardiac Conditions Requiring Prophylaxis
High-Risk Category: Prosthetic heart valves, previous endocarditis, surgical systemic pulmonary shunts
Moderate-Risk Category: Acquired valvular dysfunction (eg, rheumatic heart disease), hypertrophic cardiomyopathy, mitral valve prolapse with valvular regurgitation and/or thickened leaflets, most congenital heart malformations

125

Procedures Warranting Prophylaxis

Dental: Extractions, periodontal procedures, implants and reimplants, root canals, subgingival placement of antibiotic fibers or strips, initial placement of orthodontic bands but not brackets, intraligamentary local anesthetic injections, teeth cleaning where bleeding is expected

Respiratory Tract: Tonsillectomy and/or adenoidectomy, rigid bronchoscopy, surgery involving respiratory mucosa

GI Tract: Esophageal varices sclerotherapy, esophageal stricture dilation, endoscopic retrograde cholangiography with biliary obstruction, biliary tract surgery, surgery involving intestinal mucosa

GU Tract: Prostatic surgery, cystoscopy, urethral dilation

Cardiac Conditions Not Requiring Prophylaxis

Previous CABG surgery; mitral valve prolapse without valvular regurgitation; physiologic, functional, or innocent heart murmurs; previous rheumatic fever without valvular dysfunction; cardiac pacemakers; implanted defibrillators; isolated secundum atrial septal defect; surgical repair of atrial or ventricular septal defect

Procedures Not Warranting Prophylaxis

Dental: Restorative dentistry, local anesthetic injections, intracanal endodontic treatment, rubber dam placement, suture removal, placement of removable prosthodontic or orthodontic appliances, oral impressions, fluoride treatments, oral radiographs, orthodontic appliance adjustment

Respiratory Tract: Endotracheal intubation, flexible bronchoscopy (prophylaxis optional for high-risk patients), ear tube insertion

GI Tract: Transesophageal echocardiography, endoscopy (prophylaxis optional for high-risk patients)

GU Tract: Vaginal hysterectomy (prophylaxis optional for high-risk patients), urethral catheterization of uninfected tissue

Other: Cardiac catheterization, balloon angioplasty

Table 67. Endocarditis Prophylaxis Regimens	
Situation	**Regimen**
Dental, oral, respiratory tract, or esophageal procedures	
Standard general prophylaxis	Amoxicillin 2.0 g po 1 h before procedure
Unable to take oral medications	Ampicillin 2.0 g IM or IV ≤ 30 min before procedure
Allergic to penicillin	Clindamycin 600 mg or cephalexin 2.0 g or cefadroxil 2.0 g or azithromycin 500 mg or clarithromycin 500 mg po 1 h before procedure
Allergic to penicillin and unable to take oral medications	Clindamycin 600 mg or cefazolin 1.0 g IM or IV ≤ 30 min before procedure
GU or GI procedures	
High-risk patients	Ampicillin 2.0 g IM or IV + gentamicin 1.5 mg/kg IV or IM (not to exceed 120 mg) ≤ 30 min before procedure; 6 h later, ampicillin 1.0 g IM or IV or amoxicillin 1.0 g po

Table 67. Endocarditis Prophylaxis Regimens (cont.)	
Situation	Regimen
High-risk patients allergic to ampicillin or amoxicillin	Vancomycin 1.0 g IV over 1–2 h + gentamicin 1.5 mg/kg IV or IM (not to exceed 120 mg); complete injection or infusion ≤ 30 min before procedure
Moderate-risk patients	Amoxicillin 2.0 g po 1 h before procedure or ampicillin 2.0 g IM or IV ≤ 30 min before procedure
Moderate-risk patients allergic to ampicillin or amoxicillin	Vancomycin 1.0 g IV over 1–2 h, complete infusion ≤ 30 min before procedure

Note: See **Table 48** for details about antibiotics.
Source: Dajani AS, Taubert KA, Wilson W, et al. Prevention of bacterial endocarditis: Recommendations by the American Heart Association. *JAMA*. 1997;277:1794–1801. Copyright 1997, American Medical Association. Reprinted with permission.

Prophylaxis for Dental Patients with Total Joint Replacements (TJR)
Conditions Requiring: Inflammatory arthropathies (eg, rheumatoid arthritis, systemic lupus erythematosus); disease-, drug-, or radiation-induced immunosuppression; type 1 diabetes mellitus; first 2 yr following joint replacement; previous prosthetic joint infection; malnourishment; hemophilia
Conditions Not Requiring: Patients > 2 yr post-TJR who do not have one of the above conditions; patients with pins, plates, or screws
Dental Procedures Warranting: see those listed for endocarditis (pp 125–126)
Suggested Prophylactic Regimens: (all given 1 h before procedure)
- Not allergic to penicillin: Amoxicillin, cephalexin, or cephradine 2.0 g po
- Not allergic to penicillin and unable to take oral medications: Ampicillin 2.0 g or cefazolin 1.0 g IM or IV
- Allergic to penicillin: Clindamycin 600 mg po
- Allergic to penicillin and unable to take oral medications: Clindamycin 600 mg IV

Source: Modified from American Dental Association and American Academy of Orthopaedic Surgeons. Antibiotic prophylaxis for dental patients with total joint replacements. *JADA*. 1997;128:1004–1007. Copyright © 1997 American Dental Association. Reprinted by permission of ADA Publishing, a Division of ADA Business Enterprises, Inc.

EXERCISE PRESCRIPTION
Before Giving an Exercise Prescription
Screen patient for:
- Musculoskeletal problems: Decreased flexibility, muscular rigidity, weakness, pain, ill-fitting shoes
- Cardiac disease: Consider stress test if patient is beginning a vigorous exercise program and is sedentary with ≥ 2 cardiac risk factors (male gender, hypertension, smoking, diabetes mellitus, dyslipidemia, obesity, family history, sedentary life style).

Individualize the Prescription
Specify short- and long-term goals; include the following components:
Flexibility: Static stretching; daily, > 15 sec per muscle group
Endurance: Walking, cycling, swimming at 50%–75% of maximum HR (220 – age for men; 220 – [0.6 × age] for women); 3–4 ×/wk; goal of 20–30 min duration
Strength: Muscle resistance (weight training); 3 sets (8–15 repetitions) per muscle group 2–3 ×/wk
Balance: Tai Chi, dance, postural awareness; 1–3 ×/wk

PSYCHOTIC DISORDERS

DIAGNOSIS
Differential Diagnosis
- Bipolar affective disorder
- Delirium
- Dementia
- Drugs: eg, antiparkinsonian agents, anticholinergics, benzodiazepines or alcohol (including withdrawal), stimulants, corticosteroids, cardiac drugs (eg, digitalis), opioid analgesics
- Late-life delusional (paranoid) disorder
- Major depression
- Physical disorders: hypo- or hyperglycemia, hypo- or hyperthyroidism, sodium or potassium imbalance, Cushing's syndrome, Parkinson's disease, B_{12} deficiency, sleep deprivation, AIDS
- Pain, untreated
- Schizophrenia
- Structural brain lesions: tumor or stroke
- Seizure disorder: eg, temporal lobe

Risk Factors for Psychotic Symptoms in Elderly Persons
Chronic bed rest, cognitive impairment, female gender, sensory impairment, social isolation

MANAGEMENT
- Alleviate underlying physical causes.
- Address identifiable psychosocial triggers.
- If psychotic symptoms are severe, frightening, or may affect safety, use antipsychotic.
- Olanzapine, quetiapine, risperidone are first choice because of fewer side effects (TD extremely high in elderly patients taking typical antipsychotics [Jeste et al, *Am J Geriatr Psychiatry.* 1999;7:70–76]).

Table 68. Representative Antipsychotic Medications			
Class, Agent	**Dosage***	**Formulations**	**Comments (Metabolism)**
Atypical Antipsychotics			
Clozapine (*Clozaril*)	25–150 (1)	[T: 25, 100]	May be useful for parkinsonism and TD; sedation, orthostasis, anticholinergic, agranulocytosis, weight gain (L)
✓ Olanzapine (*Zyprexa*)	2.5–10 (1)	[T: 2.5, 5, 7.5, 10, 15, 20; disintegrating tab: 5, 10, 15, 20]	Sedation, anticholinergic effects at high doses, weight gain (L)
✓ Quetiapine (*Seroquel*)	25–800 (1–2)	[T: 25, 100, 200, 300]	Sedation, orthostasis, no dose-related EPS (L, K)

Table 68. Representative Antipsychotic Medications (cont.)			
Class, Agent	Dosage*	Formulations	Comments (Metabolism)
✓ Risperidone (*Risperdal*)	0.5–1 (1–2)	[T: 0.25, 0.50, 1, 2, 3, 4 scored; S: 1 mg/mL]	Orthostasis, EPS at high doses (L, K)
Ziprasidone (*Geodon*)	20–80 (1–2)	[C: 20, 40, 60, 80]	May increase QT$_c$; very limited geriatric data (L)
Low Potency			
Thioridazine (eg, *Mellaril*)	25–200 (1–3)	[T: 10, 15, 25, 50, 100, 150, 200; S: 30 mg/mL]	Anticholinergic, orthostasis, QT$_c$ prolongation, sedation, TD (L, K)
Intermediate Potency			
Loxapine (*Loxitane*)	2.5–20 (1–3)	[C: 5, 10, 25, 50; S: 25 mg/mL]	Anticholinergic, orthostasis, sedation, TD (L, K)
High Potency			
Haloperidol (*Haldol*)	0.5–2 (1–3); depot 100–200 mg IM q 4 wk	[T: 0.5, 1, 2, 5, 10, 20; S: 2 mg/mL; Inj: 5 mg/mL, 50 mg/mL, 100 mg/mL (depot)]	EPS, TD (L, K)

* Total mg/d (frequency/d).
Note: ✓ = preferred agents for geriatric patients.

Table 69. Management of Side Effects of Antipsychotic Medications		
Side Effect	Treatment	Comment
Drug-induced Parkinsonism	Lower dose or switch to atypical antipsychotic	Often dose related
Akathisia (motor restlessness)	Switch to atypical antipsychotic, β-blocker (eg, propranolol [*Inderal*] 20–40 mg/d) or low-dose benzodiazepine (eg, lorazepam 0.5 mg bid)	Also seen with atypical antipsychotics; more likely with traditional agents
Hypotension	Slow titration; reduce dose; change drug class	More common with low-potency agents
Sedation	Reduce dose; give at bedtime; change drug class	More common with low-potency agents
TD	Stop drug (if possible); change to atypical antipsychotic	Increased risk in elderly; may be irreversible

Note: Periodic (q 4 mo) reevaluation of antipsychotic dose and ongoing need is important (see OBRA Regulations, p 174). Older persons are particularly sensitive to side effects of antipsychotic drugs. They are also at higher risk of developing TD. Periodic use of a side-effect scale such as the AIMS (see p 168) is highly recommended.

RENAL AND PROSTATE DISORDERS

ACUTE RENAL FAILURE
Definition
An acute deterioration in renal function defined by decreased urine output or increased values of renal function tests, or both

Precipitating and Aggravating Factors
- Acute tubular necrosis due to hypoperfusion or nephrotoxins
- Medications (eg, aminoglycosides, radiocontrast materials, NSAIDs, ACE inhibitors)
- Multiple myeloma
- Obstruction (eg, BPH)
- Vascular disease (thromboembolic, atheroembolic)
- Volume depletion or redistribution of extracellular fluid (eg, cirrhosis, burns)

Evaluation
- Review medication list
- Catheterize bladder, determine postvoid residual
- Perform UA
- Perform renal ultrasonography

- Determine fractional excretion of sodium (FENa):
$$FENa = \frac{urine\ Na/plasma\ Na \times 100\%}{urine\ creatinine/plasma\ creatinine}$$
(FENa < 1% indicates prerenal cause; FENa > 3% indicates acute tubular necrosis; FENa 1%–3% is nondiagnostic.)

Treatment
- Discontinue medications that are possible precipitants; avoid contrast dyes.
- If prerenal pattern, treat CHF if present (see p 23). Otherwise, volume repletion. Begin with fluid challenge 500–1000 cc over 30–60 min. If no response, give furosemide 100–400 mg IV.
- If obstructed, leave bladder catheter in place while evaluation and specific treatment are being implemented.
- If acute tubular necrosis, monitor weights daily, record intake and output, and monitor electrolytes frequently. Fluid replacement should be equal to urinary output plus other drainage plus 500 cc/d for insensible losses.
- Dialysis is indicated when severe hyperkalemia, acidosis, or volume overload cannot be managed with other therapies or when uremic symptoms (eg, pericarditis, coagulopathy, or encephalopathy) are present.

VOLUME DEPLETION (DEHYDRATION)
Definition
Losses of sodium and water that may be isotonic (eg, loss of blood) or hypotonic (eg, nasogastric suctioning)

Precipitating Factors
- Blood loss
- Diuretics
- GI losses
- Renal or adrenal disease (eg, renal sodium wasting)
- Sequestration of fluid (eg, ileus, burns, peritonitis)

Evaluation
Clinical symptoms and signs:
- Anorexia
- Apathy, impaired mentation
- Coma (in severe dehydration)
- Nausea and vomiting
- Oliguria

- Orthostatic lightheadedness and orthostatic hypotension
- Poor skin turgor
- Shock (in severe dehydration)

- Sunken eyes
- Syncope
- Tachycardia
- Weakness
- Weight loss

Laboratory Tests
- Urine sodium (usually < 10 mEq/L) and FENa (usually < 1%)
- Serum BUN and creatinine (BUN/creatinine ratio often > 20)
- Serum electrolytes

Management
- Daily weight; monitor fluid losses and serum electrolytes, BUN, creatinine
- If mild, oral rehydration of 2–4 L of water/d and 4–8 g Na diet
- If more severe, IV 0.9% saline. Can give 1–2 liters over first hours if hemodynamically unstable, but less if there is a history of CHF.

HYPERNATREMIA
Causes
- Pure water loss:
  - insensible losses due to sweating and respiration
  - central (eg, posttraumatic, CNS tumors, meningitis) diabetes insipidus or nephrogenic (eg, hypercalcemia, lithium) diabetes insipidus
- Hypotonic sodium loss:
  - renal causes: osmotic diuresis (eg, due to hyperglycemia); postobstructive diuresis; polyuric phase of acute tubular necrosis
  - GI causes: vomiting and diarrhea, nasogastric drainage, osmotic cathartic agents (eg, lactulose)
- Hypertonic sodium gain (eg, treatment with hypertonic saline)
- Impaired thirst (eg, delirious or intubated) or access to water (eg, functionally dependent) may sustain hypernatremia

Evaluation
- Measure intake and output.
- Obtain urine osmolality:
  - > 800 mOsm/kg suggests extrarenal (if urine Na < 25 mEq/L) or remote renal water loss or administration of hypertonic Na^+ salt solutions (if urine Na > 100 mEq/L).
  - < 250 mOsm/kg and polyuria suggests diabetes insipidus.

Treatment
- Treat underlying causes.
- Correct slowly over at least 48–72 h using oral (can use pure water), nasogastric (can use pure water), or IV (D5W, $^1/_2$ or $^1/_4$ NS) fluids; correct at rate of no more than 1 mmol/L/h if acute (eg, developing over hours) and at no more than 10 mmol/L/d if of longer duration.

- Correct with normal saline only in cases of severe volume depletion with hemodynamic compromise; once stable, switch to hypotonic solution.
- When repleting, use the following formula to estimate the effect of 1 L of any infusate on serum Na:

$$\text{Change in serum Na} = \frac{\text{infusate Na} - \text{serum Na}}{\text{total body water} + 1}.$$

- Infusate Na (mmol/L): D5W = 0; $^1/_4$ NS = 34; $^1/_2$ NS = 77; NS = 154.
- Calculate total body water as a fraction of body weight (0.5 kg in older men and 0.45 kg in older women).
- Divide treatment goal (usually 10 mmol/L/d) by change in serum Na/L (from formula) to determine amount of solution to be given over 24 h.
- May need to add to compensate for ongoing obligatory fluid losses, which are usually 1.0–1.5 L/d.
- Divide amount of solution for repletion plus amount for obligatory fluid losses by 24 to determine rate per h.

HYPONATREMIA
Causes
- With increased plasma osmolality: Hyperglycemia (1.6 mEq/L decrement for each 100 mg/dL increase in plasma glucose)
- With normal plasma osmolality (pseudohyponatremia): Severe hyperlipidemia, hyperproteinemia (eg, multiple myeloma)
- With decreased plasma osmolality:
  - With extracellular fluid (ECF) excess: Renal failure, heart failure, hepatic cirrhosis, nephrotic syndrome
  - With decreased ECF volume: Renal losses from salt-losing nephropathies, diuretics, osmotic diuresis, extrarenal loss due to vomiting, diarrhea, skin losses, and third-spacing (usually urine Na $<$ 20 mEq/L, FENa $<$ 1%, and uric acid $>$ 4 mg/dL)
  - With normal ECF volume: Primary polydipsia (urine osmolarity $<$ 100 mOsm/kg), hypothyroidism, adrenal insufficiency, SIADH (urine Na $>$ 40 mEq/L and uric acid $<$ 4 mg/dL)

Management
Only if symptomatic (eg, altered mental status, seizures) or severe acute hyponatremia (eg, $<$ 120 mEq/L):
- Goal is 0.5 mEq/L/h rise in Na (more rapid correction can result in central pontine myelinolysis); time (in hours) to correct = (140 – Na)/0.5 mEq/L/h.
- Calculate free water excess (liters) = (0.5 × current body weight in kg) × (1 – [Na/140]).
- Target rate of free water removal (L/h) = free water excess/time to correct.
- Replace urine output with 3% saline or isotonic saline.
- Monitor Na closely and taper treatment when $>$ 120 or symptoms resolve.

SIADH
Definition
Hypotonic hyponatremia (< 280 mOsm/kg) with:
- Less than maximally dilute urine (usually > 100 mOsm/kg)
- Elevated urine sodium (usually > 40 mEq/L)
- Normal volume status
- Normal renal, adrenal, and thyroid function

Precipitating Factors, Causes
- Drugs (eg, SSRIs, venlafaxine, chlorpropamide, carbamazepine, NSAIDs, barbiturates)
- Neuropsychiatric factors (eg, neoplasm, subarachnoid hemorrhage, psychosis, meningitis)
- Postoperative state, especially if pain or nausea
- Pulmonary disease (eg, pneumonia, tuberculosis, acute asthma)
- Tumors (eg, lung, pancreas, thymus)

Evaluation
- BUN, creatinine, serum cortisol, TSH
- CXR
- Review of medications
- Neurologic tests as indicated
- Urine sodium and osmolality

Management
Acute Treatment: See hyponatremia management (p 132)
Chronic Treatment:
- Discontinue offending drug or treat precipitating illness.
- Restrict water to 1000–1500 mL/d.
- Liberalize salt intake.
- Demeclocycline (*Declomycin*) 150–300 mg bid [T: 150, 300] (may be nephrotoxic in patients with liver disease).

BENIGN PROSTATIC HYPERPLASIA
Evaluation (AHCPR Guidelines)
Detailed medical history focusing on the urinary tract physical examination including a digital rectal examination and a focused neurologic examination; UA; measurement of serum creatinine. Measurement of PSA is optional.

Management
Mild Symptoms: (eg, AUA score ≤ 7; see p 173) watchful waiting
Moderate to Severe Symptoms: (eg, AUA score ≥ 8; see p 173) medical or surgical treatment

Medical Treatment:*
- α-Blockers:
  - Terazosin (*Hytrin*) advance as tolerated—days 1–3, 1 mg/d at bedtime; days 4–7, 2 mg; days 8–14, 5 mg; day 15 and beyond, 10 mg [T: 1, 2, 5, 10]
  - Doxazosin (*Cardura*) start 0.5 mg with max of 16 mg/d [T: 1, 2, 4, 8]
  - Prazosin (*Minipress*) start 1 mg/d (first dose at bedtime) or bid with max 20 mg/d [T: 1, 2, 5]
  - Tamsulosin (*Flomax*) 0.4 mg half-hour after the same meal each day and increase to 0.8 mg if no response in 2–4 wk [T: 0.4]
- 5-α Reductase inhibitors:
  - Finasteride (*Proscar*) 5 mg/d [T: 5]

* Source: McConnell JD, Barry MJ, Bruskewitz RC, et al. *Benign Prostatic Hyperplasia: Diagnosis and Treatment.* Clinical Practice Guideline No. 8. Rockville, MD: Agency for Health Care Policy and Research, Public Health Service, US Dept. of Health and Human Services, February 1994. AHCPR Publication No. 94-0582.

Surgical Management (AHCPR Guidelines):
Indicated if recurrent UTI, recurrent or persistent gross hematuria, bladder stones, or renal insufficiency are clearly secondary to BPH or as indicated by symptoms, patient preference, or failure of medical treatment. Options are:
- Transurethral resection of the prostate (TURP).
- Transurethral incision of the prostate (TUIP), which is limited to prostates whose estimated resected tissue weight (if done by TURP) would be 30 g or less.
- Open prostatectomy for large glands.

PROSTATE CANCER (see p 68)

ALLERGIC RHINITIS
Definition
• The most common atopic disorder.
• Symptoms include rhinorrhea; sneezing; and irritated eyes, nose, and mucous membranes.
• May be seasonal, but in older people is more often perennial.
• Postnasal drip, mainly from chronic rhinitis, is the most common cause of chronic cough.

Therapy
Nonpharmacologic: Avoid allergens, eliminate pets and their dander, dehumidify to reduce molds; reduce outdoor exposures during pollen season; reduce house dust mites by encasing pillows and mattresses. Arachnocides reduce mites.
Pharmacologic: (see **Table 70**).
• Antihistamines reduce sneezing and rhinorrhea, not congestion; better in seasonal and allergic than perennial rhinitis; best to start before allergy season.
• Decongestants reduce nasal congestion; topical therapy is more rapid and more effective than systemic; topical use for more than a few days produces rhinitis medicamentosa (ie, rebound rhinitis). Main uses: to permit topical steroid administration; to facilitate sleep during severe attacks.
• Cromolyn works best when given before seasonal symptoms begin or before episodic exposure.
• Glucocorticoids are the most potent therapy for allergic rhinitis (reduce rhinitis, sneezing, pruritis, congestion); also effective in perennial and vasomotor rhinitis.
• Ipratropium reduces rhinitis, not congestion.
• *Neo-Synephrine,* which causes rebound rhinitis, should not be used.

Table 70. Drug Therapy for Allergic Rhinitis				
Type, Drug	Geriatric Dosage	Formu-lations	Geriatric Half-Life	Side Effects
✓ **H₁-Receptor Antagonists or Antihistamines**				
Azelastine (*Astelin*)	2 sprays bid**	[topical spray 0.1%, 100 sprays]	22–25 h	Bitter taste, nasal burning, sneezing
Cetirizine (*Zyrtec*)	5 mg/d (max)	[T: 5, 10; syrup 5 mg/mL]	Prolonged	
Fexofenadine (*Allegra, Allegra-D**)	60 mg po bid; D not recommended	[T: 30, 60, 180; C: 60]	14 h; once a day if CrCl < 40	
Loratadine (*Claritin, Claritin-D**)	5–10 mg qd; D not recommended	[T: 10; rapid-disintegrating tab 10 mg; syrup 1 mg/mL]	Metabolites > 12 d; wide variation	

(continues)

Table 70. Drug Therapy for Allergic Rhinitis (cont.)

Type, Drug	Geriatric Dosage	Formu- lations	Geriatric Half-Life	Side Effects
Chlorpheniramine (eg, *Chlor-Trimeton*)	8–12 mg bid	[T: 4, 8, 12; CT: 2; CR: 8, 12; S: 2 mg/5 mL]	20 h, longer with renal dysfunction	Sedation, dry mouth, confusion, urinary retention; dries lung secretions
Diphenhydramine (eg, *Benadryl*)	25–50 mg bid	[T: 25, 50; elixir 12.5 mg/mL]	13.5 h	Same as chlorpheniramine
Hydroxyzine (eg, *Atarax*)	25–30 mg bid	[T: 10, 25, 50]	30 h	Same as chlorpheniramine
Decongestants				
Pseudoephedrine (eg, *Sudafed*, combinations)	60 mg po q 4–6 h	[T: 30, 60; SR: 120; elixir 30 mg/5 mL]	2–16 h; varies with urine pH	Arrhythmia, insomnia, anxiety, restlessness, elevated BP
✓ Nasal Steroids				Class side effects include nasal burning, sneezing, bleeding; septal perforation (rare), fungal overgrowth (rare); no significant systemic effects
Beclomethasone (eg, *Beconase*, *Vancenase*)	1 spray bid–qid**	[topical spray 16 g (80 sprays)]	Rapid absorp- tion, hepatic metabolism	
Budesonide (eg, *Rhinocort*)	2 sprays bid or 4 qd**	[7 g (200 sprays)]		
Dexamethasone (eg, *Dexacort*)	2 sprays bid or tid**	[25 mL (200 sprays)]		
Flunisolide (eg, *Nasalide*, *Nasarel*)	2–4 sprays bid or tid**	[25 mL (200 sprays)]		
Fluticasone (eg, *Flonase*)	2 sprays qd**	[16 g (120 sprays)]		
Mometasone (*Nasonex*)	2 sprays qd**	[17 g (120 sprays)]		
Triamcinolone (eg, *Nasacort*)	2–4 sprays qd**	[10 g (100 sprays)]		
Other				
Cromolyn (*NasalCrom*)	1 spray tid–qid;** begin 1–2 wk before exposure to allergen	[2%, 4%]		Nasal irritation, headache, itching of throat
Ipratropium (*Atrovent NS*)	2 sprays bid–qid**	[0.03, 0.06%† solution]	1.6 h	Epistaxis, nasal irritation, URI, sore throat, nausea. Caution: Do not spray in eyes.

Note: ✓ = preferred for treating older persons.
Allegra-D, Claritin-D are not recommended; both also contain pseudoephedrine. Contraindicated in narrow angle glauco-ma, urinary retention, MAOI use within 14 d, severe hypertension, or CAD. May cause headache, nausea, insomnia.
** Sprays per nares.
† Use 0.06% for treatment of viral upper respiratory infection.

136

CHRONIC OBSTRUCTIVE PULMONARY DISEASE

Definition

A spectrum of chronic respiratory diseases characterized by:

- Airflow limitation
- Cough
- Dyspnea
- Frequent pulmonary infection
- Impaired gas exchange
- Sputum production

Therapy

Stepped Approach: Add steps when symptoms inadequately controlled; discontinue agent if no improvement. See **Table 71** and **Table 73**.

Smoking Cessation: Essential at any age.

Long-Term Oxygen Therapy: For indications, see **Table 74**.

MDIs: Should be used with an aerochamber; educate patients on use. Use a separate aerochamber for inhaled steroids; wash weekly; requires separate prescription.

Table 71. COPD Therapy by Severity of Symptoms		
Step Symptoms	**Therapy**	**Cautions, Comments**
1 Mild, intermittent	β₂-Agonist MDI 1–2 puffs q 2–6 h prn	Do not exceed 8–12 puffs/24 h
2 Mild to moderate, continuing	Ipratropium MDI 2–6 puffs q 6–8 h **plus** β₂-Agonist MDI 1–4 puffs qid prn or routine	Mainstay of therapy For rapid relief
3 Suboptimal response or increasing symptoms with step 2 therapy	Add theophylline-SR 200 mg bid **and/or** Albuterol-SR 4–8 mg bid **and/or** Mucokinetic agent	Or 400 mg hs for nocturnal bronchospasm **Or** at night only If sputum is very viscous
4 Persistent symptoms with step 3 therapy	Oral steroids (eg, prednisone) up to 40 mg/d for 10–14 d	With improvement, taper to lowest effective dose, alternate-day dosing, or steroid MDI With no improvement, stop steroid
5 Severe exacerbation	↑ β₂-Agonist, eg, MDI 6–8 puffs q 1/2–2 h or inhalant solution, unit dose every 1/2–2 h, **or** SC epinephrine or terbutaline, 0.1–0.5 mL, **and/or** ↑ Ipratropium MDI 6–8 puffs q 3–4 h **and** Theophylline IV **and** Methylprednisolone IV 50–100 mg STAT and q 6–8 h **and add:** Antibiotic Mucokinetic agent	 Or inhalant solution 0.5 mg q 4–8 h Calculate to bring serum level to 10–12 μg/mL Taper as soon as possible If indicated If sputum is very viscous

Source: Data in part from Standards for the diagnosis and care of patients with chronic obstructive pulmonary disease: American Thoracic Society. *Am J Respir Crit Care Med.* 1995;152 (5 Pt 2):S77–S121.

ASTHMA

Definition

Chronic inflammatory disorder of the airways; may be triggered by:

- Air pollution
- Allergens
- Chemicals
- Emotional distress
- Exercise
- Tobacco smoke
- Viruses

Characteristics

Can present at any age, but in old age: **cough** is a common presentation, it is less variable and episodic, presents more fixed obstruction, is more difficult to classify.
Symptoms:

- Chest tightness
- Cough
- Reversible and variable PEF
- Shortness of breath
- Wheezing

Therapy

Nonpharmacologic: Avoid triggers; educate patients on disease management, use of MDIs, and peak flow meters (document severity and response to therapy).
Pharmacologic: Stepped approach:

- Based on severity of symptoms.
- When symptoms controlled for 3 months, try stepwise reduction.
- If control not achieved, step up, but first review medication technique, adherence, and avoidance of triggers. (See **Table 72**, **Table 73**, **Table 74**.)

MDIs should be used with an aerochamber, and patients should be educated on their use. Use separate aerochamber for steroids; wash weekly; requires separate prescription.

Table 72. Asthma Therapy for Elderly Patients

Step 1. Mild, Intermittent Asthma

Symptom severity: Symptoms < 2/wk; night symptoms: ≤ 2/month, asymptomatic between episodes
PEF/FEV$_1$: ≥ 80% predicted; variability < 20%; normal airflow between attacks.*
Quick-relief therapy: Short-acting: inhaled β$_2$-agonist < 2/wk. Treatment depends on severity of attack. Inhaled β$_2$-agonist or cromolyn or nedocromil before exposure to trigger.
Long-term prevention: Avoid triggers. Annual influenza vaccine, pneumococcal vaccine q 6–10 yr. If using β$_2$-agonists daily or > 1 cannister/mo, step up therapy but review technique first.

Step 2. Moderate Asthma

Symptom severity: Symptoms ≥ 2/wk that affect sleep and activity.
PEF/FEV$_1$: > 60% to ≤ 80% predicted; variability 20% to 30%.
Quick-relief therapy: Short-acting: inhaled β$_2$-agonist as needed but not to exceed 3–4/d.
Long-term prevention: Daily medications: inhaled corticosteroid, 200–2000 μg preferred. Cromolyn, montelukast, nedocromil have not been studied in older people. Theophylline-SR has many interactions and side effects. If needed, add long-acting inhaled β$_2$-agonist. If there is fixed obstruction, add ipratropium.

Step 3. Severe, Persistent Asthma

Symptom severity: Continuous symptoms, limited physical activity, frequent night symptoms.
PEF/FEV$_1$: ≤ 60% predicted; variability > 30%.
Quick-relief therapy: Short-acting: inhaled β$_2$-agonist as needed for symptoms, not to exceed 3–4/d.
Long-term prevention: Daily medications: inhaled corticosteroid, 800–2000 μg or more, and either long-acting inhaled β$_2$-agonist or theophylline-SR, and/or ipratropium, and oral corticosteroid.

Table 72. Asthma Therapy for Elderly Patients (cont.)

Step 4. Severe Exacerbations

Symptom severity: Difficulty speaking sentences, walking; fingernails or lips turned blue.
Quick-relief therapy: Evaluation: ABG, ECG, CXR, serum K^+. Treat with aerosolized β_2-agonist q 20–30 min × 1 h with continuous ECG monitoring. Nasal O_2 to keep sats > 92%. Avoid theophylline or the first 4 h. Antibiotics for change in sputum. Avoid overhydration.

---

* Some degree of fixed obstruction is common in older asthmatics. To determine irreversibility, FEV_1 or PEF before and after prednisone. 0.3–1 mg/kg/d × 2 wk.

Source: Adapted from National Asthma Education and Prevention Program, *NAEPP Working Group Report: Considerations for Diagnosing and Managing Asthma in the Elderly.* Bethesda, MD: National Heart, Lung, and Blood Institute; Feb. 1996. NIH Publication No. 96-3662.

Table 73. Asthma and COPD Medications			
Drug	**Dosage**	**Half-Life**	**Side Effects (Metabolism, Excretion)**
Anticholinergics			
✓ Ipratropium (*Atrovent*)	2–6 puffs qid or 0.5 mg by nebulizer qid	2–4 h	Dry mouth, bitter taste (Lung; poorly absorbed)
Short-acting β_2-Agonists			Class side effects include tremor, nervousness, headache, palpitations, tachycardia, cough, hypokalemia. Caution: use half-doses in persons with known or suspected coronary disease (L)
✓ Albuterol (*Proventil, Ventolin*)	2–6 puffs q 4–6 h or 2.5 mg by nebulizer qid	2–7 h	
✓ Bitolterol (*Tornalate*)	1–3 puffs q 4–6 h		
Isoetharine (eg, *Bronkometer, Bronkosol*)	0.25–0.5 mL of 1% sol'n; 2 mL NS by nebulizer q 1–4 h; inhaler 1–2 puffs q 4 h		
Metaproterenol (eg, *Alupent, Metaprel*)	0.3 mL 5% sol'n q 4 h; inhaler 2–3 puffs q 3–4 h; oral forms also		
Pirbuterol (*Maxair*)*	2–3 puffs q 4–6 h	2–3 h	
Long-acting β-Agonists			Class side effects include tremor, nervousness, headache, palpitations, tachycardia, cough, hypokalemia; caution: use half-doses in persons with known or suspected coronary disease; not for acute exacerbation (L)
✓ Salmeterol (*Serevent*)	2 puffs bid	3–4 h	
Terbutaline (*Brethaire inhaler*) (*Brethine SC*) (*Brethine, Bricanyl tablets*)	2 puffs q 4–6 h 0.25 mg SC 2.5–5.0 mg tid [T: 2.5, 5]	20 h	

(continues)

Table 73. Asthma and COPD Medications (cont.)			
Drug	**Dosage**	**Half-Life**	**Side Effects (Metabolism, Excretion)**
Corticosteroids: Inhaled			Class side effects include nausea, vomiting, diarrhea, abdominal pain; oropharyngeal thrush; dosages > 1.0 mg/d may cause adrenal suppression, reduce calcium absorption and bone density, and cause bruising (L)
✓ Beclomethasone (*Beclovent, Vanceril*)	2–4 puffs bid–qid [42, 84 μg/puff, max 840 mg/d]	3 h	
✓ Budesonide (eg, *Pulmicort*)	1–2 puffs bid–qid; [100, 200, 400 μg/puff]	2–3 h	
✓ Dexamethasone (eg, *Dexacort*)	3 puffs tid–qid [100 μg/puff]	3–6 h	
✓ Flunisolide (eg, *AeroBid*)	2–4 puffs bid [250 μg/puff]	3–5 h	
✓ Fluticasone (eg, *Flovent*)	1 puff bid [44, 110, 220 μg/puff]	3 h	
✓ Triamcinolone (eg, *Azmacort*)	2 puffs tid–qid or 4 puffs bid [100 μg/puff]	2–5 h	
Corticosteroids: Oral			
Prednisone (eg, *Deltasone, Orasone*)	20 mg po bid [T: 1, 2.5, 5, 10, 20, 50; elixir 5 mg/5 mL]	3 h	Leukocytosis, thrombocytosis, sodium retention, euphoria, depression, hallucination, cognitive dysfunction; other effects with long-term use (L)
Long-acting Theophyllines			Class side effects include atrial arrhythmias, seizures, increased gastric acid secretion, ulcer, reflux, diuresis (L**)
(eg, *Quibron-T/SR*)	300–400 mg/d [T: 300 bisect, trisect tabs]	6–13 h	
(eg, *Theo-dur, Slo-Bid*)	100–200 mg po bid [T: 100, 200, 300, 450]	6–13 h	
(eg, *Uniphyl, Theo-24*)	400 mg po qd [T: 100, 200, 300, 400]	6–13 h	
Leukotriene Inhibitors			
Montelukast (*Singulair*)	10 mg po in AM [T: 10; CT: 4, 5]	2.7–5.5 h	Unknown, minimal data in elderly patients
Zafirlukast (*Accolate*)	20 mg po bid 1 h before or 2 h after meals [T: 10, 20]	10 h	Headache, somnolence, dizziness, nausea, diarrhea, abdominal pain, increased LFTs, fever (L, reduced by 50% > 65 yr) monitor coumarin anticoagulants (L)
Zileuton (*Zyflo*)	600 mg po qid [T: 600]	2.5 h	Dizziness, insomnia, nausea, abdominal pain, abnormal LFTs, myalgia (L) monitor coumarin anticoagulants (L)

Table 73. Asthma and COPD Medications (cont.)			
Drug	Dosage	Half-Life	Side Effects (Metabolism, Excretion)
Other Medications			
✓ Albuterol-Ipratropium (*Combivent*)	120 µg/21 µg, 2–3 puffs qid; 2.5 mg/ 0.5 mg by nebulizer qid	2–4 h	Same as individual agents (L, K)
Cromolyn sodium (eg, *Intal*)	2–4 puffs or 20-mg caps qid	1–2 h	Because of propellant, use MDI with caution in coronary disease or arrhythmia (L, K)
Nedocromil (*Tilade*)	2 puffs qid	2 h	Bitter taste, headache, dizziness, sore throat, cough, chest tightness (K, F)

Note: ✓ = preferred for treating older persons.
* Mechanism may be difficult for older patients to trigger.
** Clearance reduced by 30% in older patients. Caution: Initial dosage for older patients should not exceed 400 mg/d. Follow blood levels to adjust up or down for individual patients.

Table 74. Indications for Long-Term Oxygen Therapy			
Pao$_2$ Level	Sao$_2$ Level	Other	Need
≤ 55 mm Hg	≤ 88%	–	Absolute
55–59 mm Hg	≥ 89%	Signs of tissue hypoxia (ie, cor pulmonale by ECG, CHF, hematocrit > 55%)	Yes
≥ 60 mm Hg	≥ 90%	Desaturation with exercise Desaturation with sleep apnea not corrected by CPAP	Yes* Yes*

*If patient meets criteria at rest, oxygen should also be prescribed during sleep and exercise, appropriately titrated. If patient is normoxemic at rest but desaturates during exercise or sleep (Pao$_2$ ≤ 55 mm Hg), oxygen should be prescribed. Also consider CPAP or BIPAP.
Source: Data from Standards for the diagnosis and care of patients with chronic obstructive pulmonary disease: American Thoracic Society. *Am J Respir Crit Care Med.* 1995;152 (5 Pt 2):S77–S121.

COUGH

Cough is a symptom of many acute and chronic respiratory and cardiac illnesses. Therapy first identifies, then treats the underlying problem. Chronic rhinitis is the most common cause of cough in older people (see **Table 70**). For symptomatic relief of cough, the agents in **Table 75** may be helpful.

Table 75. Antitussives and Expectorants			
Drug	Dosage	Formulations	Comments (Metabolism)
Benzonatate* (*Tessalon Perles*)	100 mg po tid (max: 600 mg/d)	[C: 100, 200]	Side effects: CNS stimulation or depression, headache, dizziness, hallucination, constipation (L)
Dextromethorphan** (eg, *Benylin DM*)	10–30 mL po q 4–8 h	[C: 30; S: 10 mg/5 mL]	Side effects: mild drowsiness, fatigue (L)

(*continues*)

Table 75. Antitussives and Expectorants (cont.)

Drug	Dosage	Formulations	Comments (Metabolism)
Guaifenesin** (eg, *Robitussin*)	5–20 mL po q 4 h	[S: 100 mg/5 mL]	Side effects: none at low doses; high doses cause nausea, vomiting, diarrhea, drowsiness, abdominal pain (L)
*Histussin HC***	10 mL q 4 h up to 40 mL/d	[S: hydrocodone 2.5 mg + phenylephrine 5 mg + chlorpheniramine 2mg/mL]	Side effects: sedation, constipation, nervousness, tachycardia, hypertension, urinary retention (L)
Hydrocodone** (*Hycodan*)	5 mL po q 4–6 h	[S: 5 mg/5 mL]	Side effects include sedation, constipation, confusion (L)

Note: * = antitussive and expectorant; ** = antitussive.

PULMONARY EMBOLISM

Symptoms
Classic triad—dyspnea, chest pain, hemoptysis—occurs in $\leq$ 20% of cases. Consider PE with any of the following:
- Chest pain
- Hypotension
- Shortness of breath
- Tachycardia
- Hemoptysis
- Hypoxia
- Syncope

Diagnosis
- Ventilation-perfusion (V-P) lung scans: normal scan reduces probability of PE to 4% in a high-risk setting and effectively excludes PE in an average or low-probability setting; a high-probability scan has a sensitivity of 41% and positive predictive value of 87% in high-risk settings. With low risk of complications and a high-probability scan, begin treatment for PE; intermediate or low-probability scans are nondiagnostic and are not sufficient to exclude PE.
- D-dimer < 500 µg/L excludes PE with a nondiagnostic V-P$_R$ scan.
- Ultrasound of the lower limbs positive for DVT warrants anticoagulation without other testing.
- Spiral-chest CT has not received adequate evaluation as a noninvasive diagnostic for PE.
- Pulmonary angiography is most accurate, false negative is 0% to 10%; complication rate 5%; mortality 1–4/1000.

Pharmacologic Therapy
- Standard therapy for PE remains IV heparin followed by warfarin.
  - Heparin (see **Table 11**): mix infusion 100 units/mL in D5W; cleared through the reticuloendothelial system, half-life of anticoagulation effect 1.5 h
  - Warfarin (see p 14 and **Table 9**)
- Low-molecular-weight heparins (LMWH) appear safe and effective for both DVT and PE.
  - LMWH (see **Table 12**)
- Acute massive PE (filling defects in 2 or more lobar arteries, or the equivalent, by angiogram) associated with hypotension or severe hypoxia or high pulmonary pressures on ECG should usually be treated with thrombolytic therapy within 48 h of onset. (See **Table 12**)

SEXUAL DYSFUNCTION

IMPOTENCE (ERECTILE DYSFUNCTION)
Definition
Inability to achieve erection sufficient for intercourse. Prevalence nearly 70% by age 70.

Causes
Often multifactorial; > 50% of cases arterial, venous, or mixed vascular cause. Also:

- Diabetes mellitus
- Drug side effects
- Hyperprolactinemia
- Hypogonadism

- Neurologic: eg, disorders of the CNS, spinal cord, or PNS; autonomic neuropathy; temporal lobe epilepsy

- Psychologic: eg, depression, anxiety, bereavement
- Thyroid or adrenal disorders

Decreased bioavailable testosterone is more associated with decreased libido than with erectile dysfunction.

Evaluation
History: Type and duration of problem; relation to surgery, trauma, medication. Problems with orgasm, libido, or penile detumescence are not erectile dysfunction.
Physical:
- Neuropathy: orthostatic hypotension, impaired response to Valsalva's maneuver, absent bulbocavernosus or cremasteric reflexes
- Peyronie's disease: penile bands, plaques
- Hypogonadism: diminished male pattern hair, gynecomastia, small (< 20–25 mm long) testes
Assessment:
- Reduced penile-to-brachial pressure index suggests vascular disease.
- Cavernosometry diagnoses venous leak syndrome; reserved for surgical candidates.
- Test dose of prostaglandin E or papaverine can exclude vascular disease or confirm venous leak syndrome.
- For libido problems check total and bioavailable testosterone, LH, TSH, and prolactin.

Therapy

Table 76. Management of Erectile Dysfunction		
Cause	**Therapy**	**Comments**
Hypogonadism, poor libido	Testosterone: scrotal transdermal (*Testoderm*) [4, 6] 4–6 mg qd; or skin transdermal (*Androderm*) [2.5, 5] 5 mg/d; or testosterone cypionate or enanthate 200 mg IM q 2–4 wk or testosterone gel 1% (*Androgel*) [5 g (50 mg/24 h), 7.5 g (75 mg), 10 g (100 mg)] begin with 5 g packet qam	When given IM, can cause polycythemia, potential for increased prostate size, fluid retention, gynecomastia, liver dysfunction, but IM testosterone is inexpensive and generally well tolerated

Squeeze packet contents into palm of hand and apply, let dry; wash hands immediately. Check serum testosterone after 14 d and adjust dose; do not use in women. |

(continues)

Table 76. Management of Erectile Dysfunction (cont.)		
Cause	**Therapy**	**Comments**
Neuropathic, vascular, or mixed	Vacuum tumescence devices (*Osbon-Erec Aid, Catalyst Vacuum Device, Pos-T-Vac, Rejoyn*)	Rare: Ecchymosis, reduced ejaculation, coolness of penile tip. Good acceptance in older population; intercourse successful in 70% to 90% of cases
	Intracavernosal [5, 10, 20, 40 µg] *or* intraurethral [250, 500] prostaglandin E (*Alprostadil*)	Risks: hypotension, bruising, bleeding, priapism; erection > 4 h requires emergency treatment; intraurethral safer and more acceptable
	Penile prosthesis	Complications: infection, mechanical failure, penile fibrosis
Organic, psychogenic, or mixed	Sildenafil (*Viagra*) [25, 50, 100] start 25 mg 1 h before sexual activity; maximum 1/d	Contraindicated with use of nitrates; caution in vascular disease; least effective in vascular impotence. Several other drug interactions; metabolism reduced in liver and kidney disease, and aging. Side effects: headache, flushing, dyspepsia (mild and transient), color tinge in vision, nasal congestion, UTI, diarrhea, dizziness, and rash.

DYSPAREUNIA
Definition
Pain with intercourse.

Aggravating Factors
- Gynecologic tumors
- Interstitial cystitis
- Myalgia from overexertion during Kegel's exercises
- Osteoarthritis
- Pelvic fractures
- Retroverted uterus
- Sacral nerve root compression
- Vaginal atrophy from estrogen deprivation
- Vulvar or vaginal infection

Evaluation
- Ask about sexual problems (eg, changes in libido, partner's function, and health issues).
- Screen for depression.
- Perform pelvic examination for vulvovaginitis, vaginal atrophy, conization (decreased distensibility and narrowing of the vaginal canal), scarring, pelvic inflammatory disease, cystocele, and rectocele.

Management
- Identify and treat clinical pathology.
- Educate and counsel patients.
- Discuss hormone replacement therapy (see p 159).
- Water-soluble lubricants (eg, *Replens*) are highly effective as monotherapy for those who cannot or will not use hormones, or as a supplement to estrogen.

144

- For vaginismus (vaginal muscle spasm), trial cessation of intercourse and gradual vaginal dilation may help.
- For diminished libido, short-term use of androgens (which used long-term adversely affect health) may help; refer for counseling or sex therapy.
- For atrophic vaginitis: estrogen cream, use minimum dose (eg, 0.5 g *Premarin* [42.5 g], 2 g *Ogen* or *Estrace* [42.5 g]), daily for 2 wk, then 1–3 ×/wk thereafter; estradiol vaginal ring (*Estring*) inserted intravaginally and changed q 90 d, high degree of safety and acceptability; estradiol vaginal tablets (*Vagifem* 25 µg) inserted intravaginally daily × 2 wk, then twice/wk.

SSRI-Induced Sexual Dysfunction
- Incidence varies widely, from 1% to 20% of patients making spontaneous reports to 75% when patients are systematically questioned.
- Symptoms include anorgasmia, decreased libido, and ejaculatory dysfunction.
- Tolerance may develop up to 12 wk on treatment.
- Pharmacologic management:
  - For sertraline and citalopram (not other SSRIs), reducing dose or drug holidays (skip or reduce weekend dose) may help.
  - Adjuvant medications reported as effective for this condition in case reports include
    - Bupropion (*Wellbutrin SR, Zyban*) 75–100 mg po qd
    - Mirtazapine (*Remeron*) 15 mg po hs
    - Sildenafil (*Viagra*) 25–100 mg 1 h before intercourse

SLEEP DISORDERS

CLASSIFICATION
- Disturbance of the sleep-wake cycle
- Hypersomnolence
- Insomnia (difficulty initiating or maintaining sleep)
- Parasomnias (disorders of arousal, partial arousal, and sleep stage transition)
- Sleep apnea

SLEEP DISORDERS OTHER THAN SLEEP APNEA
Risk Factors and Aggravating Factors
Treatable Associated Medical and Psychiatric Conditions: Adjustment disorders, anxiety, bereavement, cough, depression, dyspnea (cardiac or pulmonary), GERD, nocturia, pain, paresthesias, stress

Medications That Cause or Aggravate Sleep Problems: Alcohol, antidepressants, β-blockers, bronchodilators, caffeine, clonidine, cortisone, diuretics, levodopa, methyldopa, nicotine, phenytoin, progesterone, quinidine, reserpine, sedatives, sympathomimetics including decongestants

Management
Sleep improvements are better sustained over time with behavioral treatment.
Nonpharmacologic—Measures Recommended to Improve Sleep Hygiene:
- During the daytime:
  - Get out of bed at the same time each morning regardless of how much you slept the night before.
  - Exercise daily, but not immediately before bedtime.
  - Get adequate exposure to bright light during the day.
  - Decrease or eliminate naps, unless necessary part of sleeping schedule.
  - Limit or eliminate alcohol, caffeine, and nicotine, especially before bedtime.
- At bedtime:
  - Maintain a regular sleeping time, but don't go to bed unless sleepy.
  - If hungry, have a light snack before bed (unless there are symptoms of GERD or it is otherwise medically contraindicated), but avoid heavy meals at bedtime.
  - Don't read or watch television in bed.
  - Relax mentally before going to sleep; don't use bedtime as worry time.
  - Relax before bedtime, and maintain a routine period of preparation for bed (eg, washing up and going to the bathroom).
  - Control the nighttime environment with comfortable temperature, quietness, darkness.
  - Wear comfortable bedclothes.
  - If it helps, use soothing noise, for example, a fan or other appliance or a "white noise" machine.
  - If unable to fall asleep within 15–20 min, get out of bed and perform soothing activity, such as listening to soft music or reading (but avoid exposure to bright light during these times).

Pharmacologic—Principles of Prescribing Medications for Sleep Disorders:
- Use lowest effective dose.
- Use intermittent dosing (2–4 times/ wk).
- Prescribe medications for short-term use (no more than 3–4 wk).
- Discontinue medication gradually.
- Be alert for rebound insomnia following discontinuation.

Table 77. Useful Medications for Sleep Disorders in Elderly Persons				
Class, Drug	Usual Dose	Formulations	Half-Life	Comments (Metabolism, Excretion)
Antidepressant, sedating				
Nefazodone (*Serzone*)	50–200 mg	[T: 100, 150, 200, 250]	2–4 h	Antianxiety effect; less orthostasis than with trazodone (L)
Trazodone (*Desyrel*)	25–150 mg	[T: 50, 100, 150, 300]	12 h	Moderate orthostatic effects; effective for insomnia with or without depression (L)
Benzodiazepine, intermediate-acting				
Estazolam (*ProSom*)	0.5–1.0 mg	[T: 1, 2]	12–18 h	Rapidly absorbed, effective in initiating sleep; slightly active metabolites that may accumulate (K)
Lorazepam (*Ativan*)	0.25–2 mg	[T: 0.5, 1, 2]	8–12 h	Effective in initiating and maintaining sleep; associated with falls, memory loss, rebound insomnia (K)
Temazepam (*Restoril*)	7.5–15 mg	[C: 7.5, 15, 30]	8–10 h*	Daytime drowsiness may occur with repeated use; effective for sleep maintenance; delayed onset of effect (K)
Nonbenzodiazepine, short-acting				
Zaleplon (*Sonata*)	5 mg	[C: 5, 10]	1 h	Avoid taking with alcohol or food (L)
Zolpidem (*Ambien*)	5 mg	[T: 5, 10]	1.5–4.5 h**	Confusion and agitation may occur but are rare (L)
CNS depressant, nonbarbiturate and nonbenzodiazepine				
Chloral hydrate (*Aquachloral, Supprettes*)	500–1000 mg (not to exceed 2 g as single dose or total daily dose)	[C: 500; syrup 500 mg/ 5 mL; Sp: 324, 500, 648]	8 h (active metabolite)	Hypnotic effect lost after 2 wk of continuous use; contraindicated in marked cardiac, hepatic, or renal impairment (K, L)
Hormone				
Melatonin	2–5 mg	[various]	1 h	Not regulated by FDA

* Can be as long as 30 h in elderly persons.
** 3 h in elderly persons; 10 h in those with hepatic cirrhosis.

SLEEP APNEA
Definition
Repeated episodes of apnea (cessation of airflow for $\geq$ 10 sec) or hypopnea (transient reduction [$\geq$ 50% decrease or < 50% with oxygen desaturation or an arousal] of airflow for $\geq$ 10 sec) during sleep with excessive daytime sleepiness or altered cardiopulmonary function.

Classification
Obstructive: Airflow cessation as a result of upper airway closure in spite of adequate respiratory muscle effort
Central: Cessation of respiratory effort
Mixed: Features of both obstructive and central

Associated Risk Factors, Clinical Features
Family history, hypertension, increased neck circumference, male gender, obesity, smoking, snoring, upper airway structural abnormalities (eg, soft palate, tonsils)

Evaluation
Full night's sleep study (polysomnography) in sleep laboratory indicated for those who habitually snore and either report daytime sleepiness or have observed apnea; threshold for CPAP reimbursement by Medicare is 30 apneas over a 6- to 7-h period.

Management
Nonpharmacologic:
- Use CPAP by nasal mask, nasal prongs, or mask that covers the nose and mouth (considered initial treatment for clinically important sleep apnea).
- Avoid use of alcohol or sedatives.
- Lie in lateral rather than supine position; may be facilitated by soft foam ball in a backpack.
- Lose weight (obese patients).
- Use oral appliances that keep the tongue in an anterior position during sleep or keep the mandible forward.

Pharmacologic: Beneficial mostly in mild sleep apnea.
- Protriptyline (*Vivactil*) 10–20 mg/d [T: 5, 10] L (men commonly experience urinary hesitancy or frequency and impotence)
- Fluoxetine (*Prozac*) 10–20 mg [T: 10, 20, 40; S: 20 mg/5 mL] L

Surgical:
- Tracheostomy (indicated for patients with severe apnea who cannot tolerate positive pressure or when other interventions are ineffective)
- Uvulopalatopharyngoplasty (curative in fewer than 50% of cases)
- Maxillofacial surgery (rare cases)

OTHER CONDITIONS ASSOCIATED WITH SLEEP DISORDERS

Nocturnal Leg Cramps
Stretching exercises may be helpful. Quinine, 200–300 mg po hs [T: 200, 260, 300, 325] may reduce the frequency though not the severity of leg cramps. Cinchonism, hemolysis, thrombocytopenia, and visual disturbances are notable side effects.

Restless Legs Syndrome
Diagnostic Criteria:
- Vague discomfort, usually bilateral, most commonly in calves
- Symptoms exacerbated by rest, especially at night
- Symptoms relieved by movement—jerking, stretching, or shaking of limbs; pacing

Nonpharmacologic Treatment:
- Rule out or treat iron deficiency, peripheral neuropathy.
- Avoid alcohol, caffeine, nicotine.
- If possible, avoid SSRIs, TCAs, lithium, and dopamine antagonists.
- Rub limbs.
- Use hot or cold baths, whirlpools.

Pharmacologic Treatment: Start at low dose, increase as needed:
- First line: carbidopa-levodopa (*Sinemet*) 25/100 mg, 1–2 h prior to bedtime.
- Second-line agents include dopamine agonists (see **Table 56**), carbamazepine (see **Table 57**), and gabapentin (see **Table 57**).
- For refractory cases, benzodiazepines or opioids can be tried.

Periodic Limb Movement Disorder
Diagnostic Criteria:
- Insomnia or excessive sleepiness
- Repetitive, highly stereotyped limb muscle movements (eg, extension of big toes with partial flexion of ankle, knee, and sometimes hip)
- Polysomnographic monitoring showing repetitive episodes of muscle contractions and associated arousals or awakenings
- No evidence of a medical, mental, or other sleep disorder than can account for symptoms

Treatment: Indicated for clinically significant sleep disruption or frequent arousals documented on a sleep study.
- Nonpharmacologic: cognitive-behavioral therapy
- Pharmacologic: See restless legs syndrome, above. Note: with L-dopa, patients may develop symptom augmentation that occurs earlier in the day (eg, afternoon instead of evening) and may be more severe. Treatment of augmentation may require reduction of dose or switch to dopamine agonist.

URINARY INCONTINENCE

DEFINITION
UI is not a normal part of aging. It is a loss of urine control due to a combination of
- Genitourinary pathology
- Age-related changes
- Comorbid conditions
- Environmental obstacles

CLASSIFICATION
Reversible Causes of Incontinence (DRIP Mnemonic)
Delirium
Restricted mobility (illness, injury, gait disorder, restraint)
Infection (acute, symptomatic); **I**nflammation (atrophic vaginitis); **I**mpaction of stool
Polyuria (diabetes mellitus, caffeine intake, volume overload); **P**harmaceuticals
(diuretics, autonomic agents, psychotropics)

Established Incontinence
Urge: Detrusor muscle overactivity (uninhibited bladder contractions); small to large volume loss; may be idiopathic or associated with CNS lesions or bladder irritation from infection, stones, tumors; may be associated with impaired contractility and retention (detrusor hyperactivity with impaired contractility, or DHIC).
Stress: Failure of sphincter mechanisms to remain closed during bladder filling (often due to insufficient pelvic support in women and trauma from prostate surgery in men); loss occurs with increased intra-abdominal pressure.
Overflow: Impaired detrusor contractility or bladder outlet obstruction. Impaired contractility—chronic outlet obstruction, diabetes mellitus, vitamin B_{12} deficiency, tabes dorsalis, alcoholism, or spinal disease. Outlet obstruction—in men, BPH, cancer, stricture; in women, prior incontinence surgery or large cystocele.
Mixed: Both urge and stress UI common in older women.
Functional: Inability or unwillingness to toilet because of physical, cognitive, psychologic, or environmental factors.
Other (Rare): Bladder-sphincter dyssynergia, fistulas, reduced detrusor compliance, recurrent cystitis.

RISK FACTORS
- Age-related changes (BPH, atrophic urethritis)
- CHF, nocturia, COPD, or chronic cough
- Constipation
- Dementia, depression, stroke, Parkinson's disease
- Detrusor overactivity and uninhibited contractions
- Fecal incontinence
- Increased postvoid residual or decreased bladder capacity
- Impaired ADLs
- Obesity

EVALUATION
History
- Precipitant urgency suggests detrusor overactivity.
- Loss with cough, laugh, or bend suggests stress.
- Continuous leakage suggests intrinsic sphincter insufficiency or overflow.
- Onset, frequency, volume, timing, precipitants (eg, caffeine, diuretics, alcohol, cough, medications).

Physical Examination
- Bladder distension
- Cervical cord compression (interosseus muscle wasting, Hoffmann's or Babinski's signs)
- Functional impairment (eg, mobility, dexterity)
- Mental status
- Orthostatic BP, HR
- Rectal mass or impaction
- Sacral root integrity (anal sphincter tone, anal wink, perineal sensation)
- Volume overload, edema

Male GU
Prostate consistency; symmetry; for uncircumcised, check phimosis, paraphimosis, balanitis

Female GU
Atrophic vaginitis; pelvic support (see also pp 145, 159)

Testing
Voiding Record: Record time and volume of incontinent, continent episodes; activities and time of sleep; knowing oral intake is sometimes helpful.
Standing Full Bladder Stress Test: Relax perineum and cough once—immediate loss suggests stress, several seconds' delay suggests detrusor overactivity.
Postvoid Residual: If > 100 mL, repeat; still > 100 mL suggests detrusor weakness, neuropathy, outlet obstruction, or DHIC.
Laboratory: UA and urine C&S; glucose and calcium if polyuric; renal function tests and B_{12} if urinary retention; urine cytology if hematuria or pain; PSA if cancer suspected.
Urodynamic Testing: Not routinely indicated; indicated before corrective surgery, when diagnosis is unclear, or when empiric therapy fails.

MANAGEMENT
In a stepped approach, treat all transient causes first (DRIP); avoid caffeine, alcohol, minimize evening intake of fluids.

Nonpharmacologic Behavioral Therapy (First-Line Therapy)
Detrusor Instability: Timed toileting—shortest interval to keep dry; urge control—when urgency occurs, sit or stand quietly, focus on letting urge pass, when no longer urgent walk slowly to the bathroom and void. When no incontinence for 2 d, increase voiding interval by 30–60 min until voiding every 3–4 h. Pelvic muscle exercises (see p 152).

Cognitively Impaired Persons: Prompted toileting (ask if patient needs to void) at 2- to 3-h intervals during day; encourage patients to report continence status; praise patient when continent and responds to toileting.

Stress Incontinence: Pelvic muscle (Kegel's) exercises—isolate pelvic muscles (avoid thigh, rectal, buttocks contraction); perform 3–10 sets of 10 contractions at maximum strength daily; progressively longer (up to 10-sec) contractions; follow-up and encouragement necessary; consider biofeedback for training.

Pessaries: May benefit women with vaginal or uterine prolapse.

DHIC: Treat urge first; self-intermittent clean catheterization if needed.

Pharmacologic Therapy

Estrogen replacement may benefit both detrusor instability and stress incontinence; see **Table 81** for recommended dose regimens. Topical estrogens are also effective; see p 145 for available preparations. See **Table 78** for other therapies.

Table 78. Drugs to Treat Urinary Incontinence, by Types			
R_x by UI Type	Dosage	Formulations	Comments (Metabolism)
Urge or Mixed UI*			
Dicyclomine (*Bentyl*)	10–20 mg tid	[T: 10, 20; syrup 10 mg/5 mL]	Dry mouth, blurry vision, ↑ intraocular pressure, delirium, constipation, plus postural ↓ BP, cardiac conduction disturbances (K)
Hyoscyamine (*Anaspaz, Cystospaz, Levsin*)	0.375–0.75 mg qid 0.375–0.75 po q 12 h	[T: 0.125; elixir 0.125 mg/5 mL] [SR: 0.375]	May exhibit less dry mouth, depending on dosage (K)
Imipramine (*Tofranil*)	10–50 mg qd	[T: 10, 25, 50]	Dry mouth, blurry vision, ↑ intraocular pressure, delirium, constipation, plus postural ↓ BP, cardiac conduction disturbances (L)
✓ Oxybutynin (*Ditropan, Ditropan XL*)	2.5–5.0 mg bid–tid 5–20 mg qd	[T: 5; S: 5 mg/ 5 mL] [SR: 5, 10, 15]	Dry mouth, blurry vision, ↑ intraocular pressure, delirium, constipation (L)
Propantheline (*Pro-Banthine*)	15–30 mg tid (on empty stomach)	[T: 15]	Dry mouth, blurry vision, ↑ intraocular pressure, delirium, constipation (L, K)
Flavoxate (*Urispas*)	100–200 mg tid–qid	[T: 100]	Tachycardia, palpitations, drowsiness, nervousness, nausea, vomiting, dry mouth, ↑ intraocular pressure
✓ Tolterodine (*Detrol, Detrol LA*)	2 mg bid 4 mg qd	[T: 1, 2] [C: ER 2, 4]	Dry mouth, dyspepsia, constipation (L)

Table 78. Drugs to Treat Urinary Incontinence, by Types (cont.)			
R$_x$ by UI Type	Dosage	Formulations	Comments (Metabolism)
Stress UI†			
Pseudoephedrine (many OTC, eg, *Sudafed*)	15–30 mg tid 120 mg qd, bid	[T: 30, 60; elixir 30 mg/5 mL] [SR: 120]	Headache, tachycardia, ↑ BP (L)

Note: ✓ = drugs preferred in treating older people. For prostate obstruction UI, see p 133.
* Drugs to treat urge or mixed UI: ↑ bladder capacity, ↓ involuntary contractions.
† Drugs to treat stress UI: ↑ urethral smooth muscle contraction.

Surgical Therapy
Patients with stress incontinence or intrinsic sphincter deficiency who do not respond to behavioral or pharmacologic therapy should be considered for surgery. Evaluation should include complete urodynamic studies. Case control studies indicate a cure rate of 59% to 92%, with an additional 4% to 25% improved. Complication rates vary from 6% for bulking techniques to 32% for artificial sphincters.

CATHETER CARE
- Use **only** for chronic urinary retention, nonhealing pressure ulcers in incontinent patients, and when requested by patients or families to promote comfort.
- Use closed drainage system only; avoid topical or systemic antibiotics or catheters treated with antibiotics. Silver alloy hydrogel catheters reduce UTI by 27% to 73%.
- Bacteriuria is universal; treat only if symptoms (ie, fever, inanition, anorexia, delirium), or if bacteriuria persists after catheter removal.
- Replace catheter if symptomatic bacteriuria occurs, then culture urine.
- Nursing facility patients with catheters should be kept in separate rooms.
- For acute retention catheterize for 7–10 d, then do voiding trial after catheter removal, never clamping.
- **Replacing Catheters:** Routine replacement not necessary. Changing every 4–6 wk is reasonable to prevent blockage. Patients with recurrent blockage need increased fluid intake and dilute acetic acid bladder irrigation.

VISUAL IMPAIRMENT

DEFINITION
Visual acuity 20/40 or worse; severe visual impairment (legal blindness) 20/200 or worse

EVALUATION
Acuity Testing
Near Vision: Check each eye independently with glasses using handheld Rosenbaum card at 14" or Lighthouse Near Acuity Test at 16".
Far Vision: Snellen wall chart at 20'
Visual Fields: By confrontation

Ophthalmoscopic Evaluation

Tonometry using Tonopen (portable)

Causes of Visual Impairment in Decreasing Order of Frequency
Refractive Error
Cataracts: Lens opacity on ophthalmoscopic examination. Risk factors: Age, sun exposure, smoking, corticosteroids, diabetes mellitus.
Age-Related Macular Degeneration (ARMD): Atrophy of cells in the central macular region of retinal pigmented epithelium; on ophthalmoscopic examination white-yellow patches (drusen) or hemorrhage and scars in advanced stages. Risk factors: Age, sunlight exposure, family hx, white race.
Diabetic Retinopathy: Microaneurysms, dot and blot hemorrhages on ophthalmoscopy with proliferative retinopathy ischemia and vitreous hemorrhage. Risk factors: Chronic hyperglycemia.
Glaucoma: Intraocular pressure > 21 mm Hg, optic cupping and nerve head atrophy, and loss of peripheral visual fields. Risk factors: Black race, age, family hx, elevated eye pressures.

MANAGEMENT
Prevention:
Biennial full eye examinations for persons > 65 years of age, annually for diabetic persons

Nonpharmacologic Interventions
ARMD: Photocoagulation for wet form: monitor using Amsler grid daily.
Cataract Surgery: AHCPR guidelines (AHCPR Publication No. 93-0542): if acuity 20/50 or worse with symptoms of poor functional acuity; or if 20/40 or better with disabling glare or frequent exposure to low light situations, diplopia, disparity between eyes, or occupational need; or when cataract removal will treat another lens-induced disease (eg, glaucoma); or when cataract coexists with retinal disease requiring unrestricted monitoring (eg, diabetic retinopathy)
Diabetic Retinopathy: Laser treatment of proliferative retinopathy or macular edema
Glaucoma Surgery: Open angle—laser trabeculoplasty or surgical trabeculectomy; angle closure—laser iridotomy; used primarily when pressures are poorly controlled by topical agents or when visual loss progresses
154

Pharmacologic Interventions

ARMD: Zinc oxide 80 mg, cupric oxide 2 mg, betacarotene 15 mg, vitamin C 500 mg, and vitamin E 400 IU taken in divided doses bid reduces risk of progression.

Diabetic Retinopathy: Glycemic control (see p 51)

Glaucoma: Treat when pressures are > 25 mm Hg or with optic nerve damage or visual field loss (see **Table 79**).

Table 79. Agents for Treating Glaucoma			
Drug	**Strength**	**Dosage**	**Side Effects (Metabolism)**
Adrenergic Agonists (bottles with purple caps)			
Apraclonidine (*Iopidine*)	0.5%, 1%	1–2 drops tid	Low BP, fatigue, drowsiness, dry mouth, dry nose (unknown)
Brimonidine (*Alphagan*)	0.2%	1 drop tid	Low BP, fatigue, drowsiness, dry mouth, dry nose (L)
Dipivefrin (*AKPro, Propine*)	0.1%	1 drop bid	Hypertension, headache, tachycardia, arrhythmia (eye, L)
Epinephrine (*Epifrin, Glaucon*)	0.1%–2%	1 drop qd–bid	Hypertension, headache, tachycardia, arrhythmia (L)
Epinephrine borate (*Epinal*)	0.25%–0.5%	1 drop bid	Hypertension, headache, tachycardia, arrhythmia (L)
β-Blockers (bottles with blue or yellow caps)			Class side effects: hypotension, brady-cardia, CHF, bronchospasm, anxiety, confusion, hallucination, diarrhea, nausea, cramps, lethargy, weakness, masking of hypoglycemia, impotence (L)
Betaxolol (*Betoptic, Betoptic-S*)	0.25%, 0.5%	1–2 drops bid	
Carteolol (*Ocupress*)	1%	1 drop bid	
Levobunolol (*AKBeta, Betagan*)	0.25%, 0.5%	1 drop bid	
Metipranolol (*OptiPranolol*)	0.3%	1 drop bid	
Timolol drops (*Betimol, Timoptic*)	0.25%, 0.5%	1 drop bid	
Timolol gel (*Timoptic–XE*)	0.25%, 0.5%	1 drop qd (in AM)	
Miotics, Direct-Acting (bottles with green caps)			
Pilocarpine gel (*Pilopine HS*)	4%	$^1/_2$" qhs	Systemic cholinergic effects (tissues, K)
(*Ocusert*)	20, 40 µg/h	Weekly	
Pilocarpine (*Adsorbocarpine, Akarpine, Isopto Carpine, Pilagan, Pilocar, Piloptic, Pilostat*)	0.25%–10%	1 drop qid	Systemic cholinergic effects are rare (K)

(continues)

155

Table 79. Agents for Treating Glaucoma (cont.)

Drug	Strength	Dosage	Side Effects (Metabolism)
Miotics, Cholinesterase Inhibitors (bottles with green caps)			Class side effects: cholinomimetic effects (sweating, tremor, headache, salivation), confusion, high or low BP, bradycardia, bronchoconstriction, urinary frequency, cramps, diarrhea, nausea, deterioration of mental status in persons with AD
Demecarium (*Humorsol*)	0.125%, 0.25%	1–2 drops bid	
Echothiophate (*Phospholine*)	0.03%– 0.25%	1 drop bid	
Isoflurophate (*Floropryl*)	0.025%	0.25"/8–72 h	
Physostigmine (*Eserine, Fisostin, Isopto Eserine*)	0.25% ointment	1" tid	
Carbonic Anhydrase Inhibitors (bottles with orange caps)			
Topical			Caution in renal failure (K)
✓ Brinzolamide (*Azopt*)	1%	1 drop tid	
✓ Dorzolamide (*Trusopt*)	2%	1 drop tid	
Oral			Class side effects: fatigue, weight loss, paresthesias, depression, COPD exacerbation, cramps, diarrhea, renal failure, blood dyscrasias, hypokalemia, acidosis; not recommended in renal failure (K)
Acetazolamide (eg, *Diamox*)	125–500 mg, 500 mg SR	250–500 mg bid–qid, 500 SR bid	
Dichlorphenamide (*Daranide*)	50 mg	25–50 mg qd–tid	
Methazolamide (eg, *Neptazane*)	25–50 mg	50–100 mg bid–tid	
✓ Prostaglandin Analogues			Class side effects: change in eye color and periorbital tissues, hyperemia, itching (K, L)
Bimatoprost (*Lumigan*)	0.03%	1 drop hs	
Latanoprost (*Xalatan*)	0.005%	1 drop hs	
Travoprost (*Travatan*)	0.004%	1 drop hs	
Unoprostone (*Rescula*)	0.15%	1 drop hs	
Other topical			
Dorzolamide/timolol (*Cosopt*)	0.2%, 0.05%	1 drop bid	Unusual taste, ocular itching, burning (K, L)

Note: Patients may not know names of drugs but instead refer to them by the color of the bottle cap. The usual color scheme is referenced above. ✓ = Drugs preferred for treating older people.

Low-Vision Rehabilitation and Aids
Refer patients with uncompensated visual loss causing functional deficits. Aids include optical, nonoptical, low- and high-technology devices. Strategies include improved illumination, increased contrast, magnification, and auditory and tactile feedback. Environmental modifications include using color contrast, floor lamps to reduce glare, motion sensors to turn on lights, high-technology options including video magnification with closed-circuit television and word processing programs to enlarge text.

Acute Conjunctivitis
Symptoms: Red eye, foreign body sensation, discharge, photophobia
Signs: Conjunctival hyperemia and discharge. Visual acuity, pupillary light reflexes, and visual fields are normal. If eye functions are abnormal, refer to ophthalmology for urgent diagnosis.
Differential diagnosis: Acute iritis, acute glaucoma, episcleritis, or scleritis.
Etiology: **Viral**, bacterial, chlamydial, chemical, foreign body
Viral versus bacterial: **Viral**—profuse tearing, minimal exudation, preauricular adenopathy common, monocytes in stained scrapings and exudates; **bacterial**—moderate tearing, profuse exudation, preauricular adenopathy uncommon, bacteria and polymorphonuclear cells in stained scrapings and exudates; **both**—minimal itching, generalized hyperemia, occasional sore throat and fever.
Treatment: Majority are viral; treat symptoms with artificial tears and cool compresses. If purulent discharge, suspect bacterial; start broad-spectrum topical antibiotics (see **Table 80**). If severe, obtain culture and Gram's stain, then start treatment. If signs and symptoms fail to improve in 24–48 h, refer to ophthalmologist. If vision decreased or severe pain, refer to ophthalmologist immediately.
Other: Frequent hand washing and use of separate towels to avoid spread

Table 80. Treatment for Acute Bacterial Conjunctivitis*		
Agent	**Formulations****	**Comment**
Ciprofloxacin (*Ciloxan Ophthalmic*)	0.3% solution, 0.3% ointment	Very broad spectrum, well tolerated, a 1st choice in severe cases, expensive
Erythromycin ophthalmic (*AK-Mycin, Ilotycin*)	5 mg/gm ointment	Good if staphylococcal blepharitis is present
Norfloxacin (*Chibroxin*)	0.3% solution	Very broad spectrum, well tolerated, a 1st choice in severe cases, expensive
Ofloxacin (*Floxin, Ocuflox Ophthalmic*)	0.3% solution, 0.3% ointment	Very broad spectrum, well tolerated, a 1st choice in severe cases, expensive
Sulfacetamide sodium (*Sodium Sulamyd*)	10%, 30% drops, 10% ointment	Same coverage as trimethoprim and polymyxin
Tobramycin (*AKTob, Tobrex*)	3 mg/gm ointment, 3 mg/mL solution	Well tolerated, but more corneal toxic
Trimethoprim and polymyxin (*Polytrim*)	1 mg/mL, 10,000 IU/mL solution	Well tolerated but some gaps in coverage

* Do not use steroid or steroid-antibiotic preparations in initial treatment.
** In mild cases solution is applied qid and gel or ointments bid for 5–7 d. In more severe cases solution is applied q 2–3 h, ointment qid; as the eye improves, solution is applied qid and ointment, bid.

PREVENTION
• Annual breast and pelvic and perineal examination
• Annual mammography as appropriate
• Discuss hormone replacement therapy
• One negative Pap smear after 65 yr if low risk (ie, single established sexual partner, good prior screening, no hx of abnormal Pap smear or genital herpes)
• Osteoporosis evaluation (see p 105)

COMMON DISORDERS
Vulvar Diseases
Non-neoplastic:
• Lichen sclerosus—Occurs commonly on vulva of middle-aged and older women; causes 1/3 of benign vulvar lesions, extends to perirectal areas (classic hourglass appearance); lesions are white to pink macules or papules, may coalesce; symptoms are none or itching, soreness, or dyspareunia. Must biopsy for diagnosis.
  R_x: Petrolatum or testosterone propionate 2% or clobetasol propionate 0.05% qd–bid for 6–12 wk; if symptoms resolve, switch to hydrocortisone 1% prn.
• Squamous hyperplasia—Raised white keratinized lesions difficult to distinguish from vulvar intraepithelial neoplasia (VIN); must biopsy to exclude malignancy.
  R_x: Betamethasone dipropionate 0.05% for 6–8 wk, then 1% hydrocortisone if symptoms persist.

Neoplastic:
• VIN—Most often seen in postmenopausal women; asymptomatic or may cause pruritus; appear as hypo- or hyperpigmented keratinized lesions; often multifocal; inspection ± colposcopy of the entire vulva with biopsy of most worrisome lesions; lesions graded on degree of atypia. R_x: surgical or other ablative therapy.
• Vulvar malignancy—Half of cases occur in women aged > 70 yr; 80% are squamous cell, with melanoma, sarcoma, basal cell, and adenocarcinoma < 20%; biopsy any suspicious lesion. R_x: radical surgery is preferred treatment.

Postmenopausal Bleeding
Bleeding after 1 yr of amenorrhea:
• Exclude malignancy, identify source, treat symptoms.
• Examine genitalia, perineum, rectum.
• If endometrial source, use endometrial biopsy or vaginal probe ultrasound to assess endometrial thickness (< 5 mm virtually excludes malignancy).
• D&C when endometrium not otherwise adequately assessed.
• Women on combination continuous estrogen and progesterone who bleed after 12 mo need evaluation.
• Those on cyclic replacement with bleeding at unexpected times (ie, bleeding other than during the second week of progesterone therapy) need evaluation.

Hot Flushes

- Vasomotor symptoms respond to estrogen (see **Table 81**) in dos
  start low dose, titrate to effect.
- If estrogen cannot be taken, try one of the less effective alterna
  - megestrol (*Megace*): [T: 20, 40] 20 mg bid
  - medroxyprogesterone acetate (eg, *Cycrin, Provera*): [T: 2.5, 5,
  - clonidine (*Catapres, Duraclon*): [T: 0.1, 0.2, 0.3] 0.1–0.3 mg/d

Vaginal Prolapse

- Child-bearing and other causes of increased intra-abdominal pressure weaken connective tissue and muscles supporting the genital organs, leading to prolapse.
- Symptoms include: Pelvic pressure, back pain, fecal or urinary incontinence, difficulty evacuating the rectum. Symptoms may be present even with mild prolapse.
- The degree of prolapse and organs involved dictate therapy; no therapy if asymptomatic.
- Estrogen and Kegel's exercises may help in mild cases.
- Pessary or surgery indicated with greater symptoms. Surgery needed for 4th- degree symptomatic prolapse.
- Precise anatomic defect(s) dictates the surgical approach.
- A common (ACOG) classification for degrees of prolapse:
  - First degree—extension to the mid-vagina
  - Second degree—approaching the hymenal ring
  - Third degree—at the hymenal ring
  - Fourth degree—beyond the hymenal ring

Atrophic Vaginitis (See p 145)

Hormone Replacement Therapy

Estrogen Replacement: After menopause, associated with preservation of bone mass. Effects on cardiovascular risk and cognitive capacity are uncertain. May increase risk of coronary events during first 1–2 yr of therapy in women with CAD. Positive effects on urogenital health include reduced dyspareunia, maintenance of continence, and reduction in urinary tract infections.

- When the patient has a uterus, estrogen should be combined with progesterone to reduce endometrial cancer risk.
- Some women prefer unopposed estrogen and annual biopsy. Common regimens are given in **Table 81**.

Estrogen Risks, Side Effects: Estrogen therapy increases risk of endometrial cancer, risk that is attenuated or eliminated by progestational agents.

- Breast cancer risk increased by higher dose and with ≥ 5 yr of use.
- Risks also include thromboembolism and gallbladder disease.
- Ovarian cancer risk may be increased with > 10 yr of use.

Contraindications:

- Undiagnosed vaginal bleeding
- Active thromboembolic disease
- Probably breast cancer
- Endometrial cancer greater than stage 1
- Possibly gallbladder disease
- Menstrual migraine

Table 81. Common Regimens for Hormone Replacement Therapy

	Starting Dosage (mg/d)	Cyclic Dosing	Continuous Dosing	Formulations
...ugated equine ...trogen (*Premarin*)*	0.3–0.625	—	Daily	[T: 0.3, 0.625, 0.9, 1.25, 2.5]
Conjugated synthetic estrogen (*Cenestin*)	0.625	—	Daily	[T: 0.625, 0.9, 1.25]
Esterified estrogen (eg, *Estratab, Menest*)*	0.3–0.625	—	Daily	[T: 0.3, 0.625, 1.25, 2.5]
Estropipate (*Ogen, Ortho-Est*)*	0.625	—	Daily	[T: 0.625, 1.25, 2.5]
Micronized 17-β estradiol (*Estrace*)*	0.5–1.0	—	Daily	[T: 0.5, 1, 2]
Transdermal estrogen				
(*Alora*)	0.05–0.75	—	Biweekly	[0.05 0.075, 0.1]
(*Estraderm*)*	0.05–0.75		Biweekly	[0.05, 0.1]
(*Vivelle*)*	0.0375–0.05		Biweekly	[0.025, 0.0375, 0.05, 0.075, 0.1]
(*Climara*)*	0.025–0.05	—	Weekly	[0.025, 0.05, 0.075, 0.1]
(*FemPatch*)	0.025–0.05	—	Weekly	[0.025]
Estradiol *and* norethindrone (*CombiPatch*)	0.05/0.14	Biweekly for 3 wk, 1 wk off	—	[0.05/0.14, 0.05/0.25]
Medroxyprogesterone (*Cycrin, Provera*)	2.5–10.0	5–10 mg, days 1–14	2.5–5 mg daily	[T: 2.5, 5, 10]
Combinations				
Conjugated estrogen *and*	0.625	—	Daily	[Fixed dose 0.625/2.5 or 0.625/5.0]
medroxyprogesterone (*Prempro* 2.5, *Prempro* 5.0 mg)	2.5, 5.0			
Conjugated estrogen *and*	0.625	Days 1–28	—	[Fixed dose 0.625 days 1–14, 0.625/5.0 days 15–28]
medroxyprogesterone (*Premphase*)	5.0	Days 15–28		
Estradiol *and*	1.0	—	Daily	[Fixed dose 1.0/5.0]
norethindrone (*FEMHRT 1/5*)	5.0			

* FDA approved for long-term use to prevent osteoporosis.

160

MINI-COG ASSESSMENT INSTRUMENT FOR DEMENTIA

The Mini-Cog assessment instrument combines an uncued 3-item recall test with a clock-drawing test (CDT). The Mini-Cog can be administered in about 3 minutes, requires no special equipment, and is relatively uninfluenced by level of education or language variations.

Administration
The test is administered as follows:

1. Instruct the patient to listen carefully to 3 unrelated words and then to repeat the words.

2. Instruct the patient to draw the face of a clock, either on a blank sheet of paper, or on a sheet with the clock circle already drawn on the page.

   After the patient puts the numbers on the clock face, ask him or her to draw the hands of the clock to read a specific time, such as 11:20. These instructions can be repeated, but no additional instructions should be given. Give the patient as much time as needed to complete the task. The CDT serves as the recall distractor.

3. Ask the patient to repeat the 3 previously presented words.

Scoring
Give 1 point for each recalled word after the CDT distractor. Score 1–3.

The CDT is considered normal if all numbers are present in the correct sequence and position, and the hands readably display the requested time.

See Mini-Cog Scoring Algorithm on next page.

MINI-COG SCORING ALGORITHM

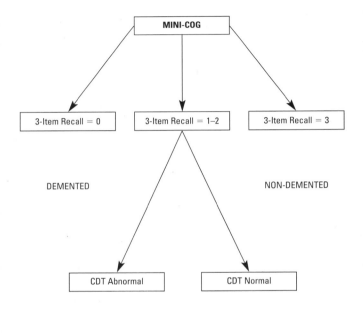

Source: Borson S, Scanlan J, Brush M, Vitaliano P, Dokmak A. The mini-cog: a cognitive "vital signs" measure for dementia screening in multi-lingual elderly. *Int J Geriatr Psychiatry* 2000; 15(11): 1021–1027. Copyright John Wiley & Sons, Ltd. Reprinted with permission.

PHYSICAL SELF-MAINTENANCE SCALE
(ACTIVITIES OF DAILY LIVING, OR ADLs)

In each category, circle the item that most closely describes the person's highest level of functioning and record the score assigned to that level (either 1 or 0) in the blank at the beginning of the category.

A. Toilet
    1. Care for self at toilet completely; no incontinence 1
    2. Needs to be reminded, or needs help in cleaning self, or has rare
       (weekly at most) accidents 0
    3. Soiling or wetting while asleep more than once a week 0
    4. Soiling or wetting while awake more than once a week 0
    5. No control of bowels or bladder 0

B. Feeding
    1. Eats without assistance 1
    2. Eats with minor assistance at meal times and/or with special
       preparation of food, or help in cleaning up after meals 0
    3. Feeds self with moderate assistance and is untidy 0
    4. Requires extensive assistance for all meals 0
    5. Does not feed self at all and resists efforts of others to feed him or her 0

C. Dressing
    1. Dresses, undresses, and selects clothes from own wardrobe 1
    2. Dresses and undresses self, with minor assistance 0
    3. Needs moderate assistance in dressing and selection of clothes. 0
    4. Needs major assistance in dressing, but cooperates with efforts of
       others to help 0
    5. Completely unable to dress self and resists efforts of others to help 0

D. Grooming (neatness, hair, nails, hands, face, clothing)
    1. Always neatly dressed, well-groomed, without assistance 1
    2. Grooms self adequately with occasional minor assistance, eg, with shaving 0
    3. Needs moderate and regular assistance or supervision with grooming 0
    4. Needs total grooming care, but can remain well-groomed after help from others .. 0
    5. Actively negates all efforts of others to maintain grooming 0

E. Physical Ambulation
    1. Goes about grounds or city 1
    2. Ambulates within residence on or about one block distant 0
    3. Ambulates with assistance of (check one)
       a ( ) another person, b ( ) railing, c ( ) cane, d ( ) walker, e ( ) wheelchair 0
       1.__ Gets in and out without help. 2.__ Needs help getting in and out.
    4. Sits unsupported in chair or wheelchair, but cannot propel self without help ... 0
    5. Bedridden more than half the time 0

F. Bathing
    1. Bathes self (tub, shower, sponge bath) without help. 1
    2. Bathes self with help getting in and out of tub. 0
    3. Washes face and hands only, but cannot bathe rest of body. 0
    4. Does not wash self, but is cooperative with those who bathe him or her. 0
    5. Does not try to wash self and resists efforts to keep him or her clean. 0

For scoring interpretation and source, see note following the next instrument.

INSTRUMENTAL ACTIVITIES OF DAILY LIVING SCALE (IADLs)

In each category, circle the item that most closely describes the person's highest level of functioning and record the score assigned to that level (either 1 or 0) in the blank at the beginning of the category.

A. Ability to Use Telephone _____
1. Operates telephone on own initiative; looks up and dials numbers. 1
2. Dials a few well-known numbers. 1
3. Answers telephone, but does not dial. 1
4. Does not use telephone at all. 0

B. Shopping _____
1. Takes care of all shopping needs independently. 1
2. Shops independently for small purchases. 0
3. Needs to be accompanied on any shopping trip. 0
4. Completely unable to shop. 0

C. Food Preparation _____
1. Plans, prepares, and serves adequate meals independently. 1
2. Prepares adequate meals if supplied with ingredients. 0
3. Heats and serves prepared meals or prepares meals, but does not
   maintain adequate diet. 0
4. Needs to have meals prepared and served. 0

D. Housekeeping _____
1. Maintains house alone or with occasional assistance (eg, heavy-
   work domestic help). 1
2. Performs light daily tasks such as dishwashing, bedmaking. 1
3. Performs light daily tasks, but cannot maintain acceptable level of
   cleanliness. 1
4. Needs help with all home maintenance tasks. 1
5. Does not participate in any housekeeping tasks. 0

E. Laundry _____
1. Does personal laundry completely. 1
2. Launders small items; rinses socks, stockings, etc. 1
3. All laundry must be done by others. 0

F. Mode of Transportation _____
1. Travels independently on public transportation or drives own car. 1
2. Arranges own travel via taxi, but does not otherwise use public
   transportation. 1
3. Travels on public transportation when assisted or accompanied
   by another. 1
4. Travel limited to taxi or automobile with assistance of another. 0
5. Does not travel at all. 0

G. Responsibility for Own Medications _____
1. Is responsible for taking medication in correct dosages at correct time. 1
2. Takes responsibility if medication is prepared in advance in separate
   dosages. 0
3. Is not capable of dispensing own medication. 0

H. Ability to Handle Finances _____

1. Manages financial matters independently (budgets, writes checks,
   pays rent and bills, goes to bank); collects and keeps track of income. 1
2. Manages day-to-day purchases, but needs help with banking,
   major purchases, etc. 1
3. Incapable of handling money. 0

Scoring Interpretation: For ADLs, the total score ranges from 0 to 6, and for IADLs, from 0 to 8. In some categories, only the highest level of function receives a 1; in others, two or more levels have scores of 1 because each describes competence that represents some minimal level of function. These screens are useful for indicating specifically how a person is performing at the present time. When they are also used over time, they serve as documentation of a person's functional improvement or deterioration.

Source: Republished with permission from Lawton MP, Brody EM. Assessment of older people: self-maintaining and instrumental activities of daily living. Gerontologist 1969;9:179–186. Permission conveyed through Copyright Clearance Center, Inc..

GERIATRIC DEPRESSION SCALE (GDS, SHORT FORM)

Choose the best answer for how you felt over the past week.

1. Are you basically satisfied with your life?		yes/**no**
2. Have you dropped many of your activities and interests?		**yes**/no
3. Do you feel that your life is empty?		**yes**/no
4. Do you often get bored?		**yes**/no
5. Are you in good spirits most of the time?		yes/**no**
6. Are you afraid that something bad is going to happen to you?		**yes**/no
7. Do you feel happy most of the time?		yes/**no**
8. Do you often feel helpless?		**yes**/no
9. Do you prefer to stay at home, rather than going out and doing new things?		**yes**/no
10. Do you feel you have more problems with memory than most?		**yes**/no
11. Do you think it is wonderful to be alive now?		yes/**no**
12. Do you feel pretty worthless the way you are now?		**yes**/no
13. Do you feel full of energy?		yes/**no**
14. Do you feel that your situation is hopeless?		**yes**/no
15. Do you think that most people are better off than you are?		**yes**/no

Score 1 point for each **bolded** answer. Cut-off: normal (0–5), above 5 suggests depression.

Source: Courtesy of Jerome A. Yesavage, MD. For 30 translations of the GDS, see
http://www.stanford.edu/~yesavage/GDS.html
For additional information on administration and scoring refer to the following references:
1. Sheikh JI, Yesavage JA. Geriatric Depression Scale: recent evidence and development of a shorter version. *Clin Gerontol.* 1986;5:165–172.
2. Feher EP, Larrabee GJ, Crook TH 3rd. Factors attenuating the validity of the Geriatric Depression Scale in a dementia population. *J Am Geriatr Soc.* 1992;40:906–909.
3. Yesavage JA, Brink TL, Rose TL, et al. Development and validation of a geriatric depression rating scale: a preliminary report. *J Psychiatr Res.* 1983;17:27.

BRIEF HEARING LOSS SCREENER

Points

1. Age:_____
   If age > 70 years = 1 point   _____

2. Sex: Male_____ Female_____   _____
   If male = 1 point

3. Highest grade attended: _____
   12th grade or less _____
   higher than 12th grade_____
   If ≤ 12th grade = 1 point

4. Have you ever had deafness or trouble hearing with one or both ears?   __0__
   Yes _____, continue to Question #5.
   No _____, go to Question #6.
   No points assigned to this question.

5. Did you ever see a doctor about it?   _____
   Yes_____ No_____
   If "Yes" = 2 points

6. Without a hearing aid, can you usually hear and understand what a person   _____
   says without seeing his/her face if that person whispers to you
   from across the room?
   Yes_____ No_____
   If "No" = 1 point

7. Without a hearing aid, can you usually hear and understand what a person   _____
   says without seeing his/her face if that person talks to you in a normal voice
   from across the room?
   Yes_____ No_____
   If "No" = 2 points

TOTAL   _____

3 or more points is a positive score indicating the need for further evaluation.

	Sensitivity	Specificity	Pos Predictive Value	Neg Predictive Value
Ventry-Weinstein criteria	80%	80%	45%	95%
High-frequency pure-tone average	59%	88%	76%	77%

Source: Reuben DB, Walsh K, Moore AA, et al. Hearing loss in community-dwelling older persons: national prevalence data and identification using simple questions. *J Am Geriatr Soc.* 1998;46:1011. Reprinted with permission.

PERFORMANCE-ORIENTED MOBILITY ASSESSMENT (POMA)

Balance

Chair: Instructions: Place a hard armless chair against a wall. The following maneuvers are tested.

1. Sitting down
    0 = unable without help or collapses (plops) into chair *or* lands off center of chair
    1 = able and does not meet criteria for 0 or 2
    2 = sits in a smooth, safe motion *and* ends with buttocks against back of chair and thighs centered on chair

2. Sitting balance
    0 = unable to maintain position (marked slide forward or leans forward or to side)
    1 = leans in chair slightly or slight increased distance from buttocks to back of chair
    2 = steady, safe, upright

3. Arising
    0 = unable without help or loses balance or requires > three attempts
    1 = able but requires three attempts
    2 = able in ≤ two attempts

4. Immediate standing balance (first 5 seconds)
    0 = unsteady, marked staggering, moves feet, marked trunk sway or grabs object for support
    1 = steady but uses walker or cane or mild staggering but catches self without grabbing object
    2 = steady without walker or cane or other support

Stand

5a. Side-by-side standing balance
    0 = unable *or* unsteady *or* holds ≤ 3 seconds
    1 = able *but* uses cane, walker, or other support *or* holds for 4–9 seconds
    2 = narrow stance without support for 10 seconds

5b. Timing ___ ___ . ___ seconds

6. Pull test (person at maximum position attained in #5, examiner stands behind and exerts mild pull back at waist)
    0 = begins to fall
    1 = takes more than two steps back
    2 = fewer than two steps backward and steady

7a. Able to stand on right leg unsupported
    0 = unable *or* holds onto any objects *or* able for < 3 seconds
    1 = able for 3 or 4 seconds
    2 = able for 5 seconds

7b. Timing ___ ___ . ___ seconds

8a. Able to stand on left leg unsupported
    0 = unable *or* holds onto any object *or* able for < 3 seconds
    1 = able for 3 or 4 seconds
    2 = able for 5 seconds

8b. Timing ___ ___ . ___ seconds

9a. Semitandem stand
    0 = unable to stand with one foot half in front of other with feet touching *or* begins to fall *or* holds for ≤ 3 seconds
    1 = able for 4 to 9 seconds
    2 = able to semitandem stand for 10 seconds

9b. Timing ___ ___ . ___ seconds

10a. Tandem stand
    0 = unable to stand with one foot in front of other *or* begins to fall *or* holds for ≤ 3 seconds
    1 = able for 4 to 9 seconds
    2 = able to tandem stand for 10 seconds

10b. Timing ___ ___ . ___ seconds

11. Bending over (to pick up a pen off floor)
    0 = unable *or* is unsteady
    1 = able, but requires more than one attempt to get up
    2 = able and is steady
12. Toe stand
    0 = unable
    1 = able but < 3 seconds
    2 = able for 3 seconds
13. Heel stand
    0 = unable
    1 = able but < 3 seconds
    2 = able for 3 seconds

Gait: Instructions: Person stands with examiner, walks down 10-ft walkway (measured). Ask the person to walk down walkway, turn, and walk back. The person should use customary walking aid.

Bare Floor (flat, even surface)
1. Type of surface: 1 = linoleum or tile; 2 = wood; 3 = cement or concrete; 4 = other
   _____ [not included in scoring]
2. Initiation of gait (immediately after told to "go")
    0 = any hesitancy or multiple attempts to start
    1 = no hesitancy
3. Path (estimated in relation to tape measure). Observe excursion of foot closest to tape
   measure over middle 8 feet of course.
    0 = marked deviation
    1 = mild or moderate deviation *or* uses walking aid
    2 = straight without walking aid
4. Missed step (trip or loss of balance)
    0 = yes, and would have fallen *or* more than two missed steps
    1 = yes, but appropriate attempt to recover *and* no more than two missed steps
    2 = none
5. Turning (while walking)
    0 = almost falls
    1 = mild staggering, but catches self, uses walker or cane
    2 = steady, without walking aid
6. Step over obstacles (to be assessed in a separate walk with two shoes placed on course
   4 feet apart)
    0 = begins to fall at any obstacle *or* unable *or* walks around any obstacle *or* > two missed
        steps
    1 = able to step over all obstacles, but some staggering and catches self *or* one to two
        missed steps
    2 = able and steady at stepping over all four obstacles with no missed steps

Source: Courtesy of Mary E. Tinetti, MD. Adapted with permission.

ABNORMAL INVOLUNTARY MOVEMENT SCALE (AIMS)

Examination Procedure
Either before or after completing the examination procedure, observe the patient
unobtrusively, at rest (eg, in waiting room).

The chair to be used in this examination should be a hard, firm one without arms.

1. Ask patient to remove shoes and socks.
2. Ask patient whether there is anything in his/her mouth (ie, gum, candy, etc) and if
   there is, to remove it.

3. Ask patient about the **current** condition of his/her teeth. Ask patient if he/she wears dentures. Do teeth or dentures bother patient **now**?
4. Ask patient whether he/she notices any movements in mouth, face, hands, or feet. If yes, ask to describe and to what extent they **currently** bother patient or interfere with his/her activities.
5. Have patient sit in chair with hands on knees, legs slightly apart, and feet flat on floor. (Look at entire body for movements while in this position.)
6. Ask patient to sit with hands hanging unsupported. If male, between legs, if female and wearing a dress, hanging over knees. (Observe hands and other body areas.)
7. Ask patient to open mouth. (Observe tongue at rest within mouth.) Do this twice.
8. Ask patient to protrude tongue. (Observe abnormalities of tongue movement.) Do this twice.
9. Ask patient to tap thumb with each finger as rapidly as possible for 10–15 seconds; separately with right hand, then with left hand. (Observe facial and leg movements.)
10. Flex and extend patient's left and right arms (one at a time). (Note any rigidity.)
11. Ask patient to stand up. Observe in profile. Observe all body areas again, hips included.)
12. Ask patient to extend both arms outstretched in front with palms down. (Observe trunk, legs, and mouth.)
13. Have patient walk a few paces, turn, and walk back to chair. (Observe hands and gait.) Do this twice.

Instructions: Complete examination procedure before making ratings. Rate highest severity observed.
Code:
   1 None
   2 Minimal, may be extreme normal
   3 Mild
   4 Moderate
   5 Severe

Facial and Oral Movements
1. Muscles of facial expression (eg, movements of forehead, eyebrows, periorbital area, cheeks; including frowning, blinking, smiling, grimacing)

1	2	3	4	5

2. Lips and perioral area (eg, puckering, pouting, smacking)

1	2	3	4	5

3. Jaw (eg, biting, clenching, chewing, mouth opening, lateral movement)

1	2	3	4	5

4. Tongue (rate only increase in movement both in and out of mouth, NOT inability to sustain movement)

1	2	3	4	5

Extremity Movements
5. Upper (arms, wrists, hands, fingers). Include choreic movements (ie, rapid, objectively purposeless, irregular, spontaneous), athetoid movements (ie, slow, irregular, complex, serpentine). Do NOT include tremor (ie, repetitive, regular, rhythmic).

1	2	3	4	5

6. Lower (legs, knees, ankles, toes). (Eg, lateral knee movement, foot tapping, heel dropping, foot squirming, inversion and eversion of foot)

1	2	3	4	5

Trunk Movements
7. Neck, shoulders, hips (eg, rocking, twisting, squirming, pelvic gyrations)

1	2	3	4	5

Global Judgments

8. Severity of abnormal movements
   1 None, normal
   2 Minimal
   3 Mild
   4 Moderate
   5 Severe

9. Incapacitation due to abnormal movements
   1 None, normal
   2 Minimal
   3 Mild
   4 Moderate
   5 Severe

10. Patient's awareness of abnormal movements (rate only patient's report)
    1 No awareness
    2 Aware, no distress
    3 Aware, mild distress
    4 Aware, moderate distress
    5 Aware, severe distress

Dental Status

11. Current problems with teeth and/or dentures
    1 No
    2 Yes

12. Does patient usually wear dentures?
    1 No
    2 Yes

Source: Adapted from Department of Health and Human Services, Public Health Service, Alcohol, Drug Abuse and Mental Health Administration, National Institute of Mental Health. *Treatment Strategies in Schizophrenia Study.* ADM-117. Revised 1985.

PAIN SCALES FOR ASSESSING PAIN INTENSITY

Use copies of pain scales that are large enough for older patients to see comfortably (14-point font or larger).

Faces Pain Scale

Place an X under the face that best represents the severity or intensity of your pain right now.

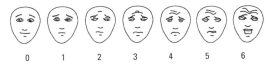

    0   1   2   3   4   5   6

Source: Reprinted from *Pain*, 41(2), Bien D, Reeve R, Champion G, et al. The Faces Pain Scale for the self-assessment of the severity of pain experienced by children: development and initial validation, and preliminary investigation for ratio scale properties. 139–150, Copyright 1990, with permission from Elsevier Science.

0–10 Numeric Rating Scales

Verbal: On a scale of 0–10, with 0 being no pain and 10 being the most intense pain imaginable, what would you rate the severity or intensity of your pain right now? _____

Source: Keela Herr, 1999.

Visual: Circle the number that best represents the severity or intensity of your pain right now.

0	1	2	3	4	5	6	7	8	9	10
No pain					Moderate pain					Worst possible pain

Source: Carr DB, Jacox AK, Chapman CR, et al. *Acute Pain Management: Operative Medical Procedures and Trauma.*
Clinical Practice Guideline No. 1. Rockville, MD: AHCPR, Public Health Service, US Dept of Health and Human Services;
February 1992. AHCPR Publication No. 92-0032.

Verbal Descriptor Scale

Place an X beside the words that best describe the severity or intensity of your pain right now. Mark one set of words.

_____ The Most Intense Pain Imaginable
_____ Very Severe Pain
_____ Severe Pain
_____ Moderate Pain
_____ Mild Pain
_____ Slight Pain
_____ No Pain

Source: Keela Herr, 1999.

References
AGS Panel on Chronic Pain in Older Persons. The management of chronic pain in older persons. *J Am Geriatr Soc.*
1998;46:635–651.
Herr KA, Mobiliy PR, Kohout FJ, et al. Evaluation of the faces pain scale for use with the elderly. *Clin J Pain.*
1998;14:29–38.

10-MINUTE SCREENER FOR GERIATRIC CONDITIONS

Problem	Screening Measure	Positive Screen
Vision	Two parts: Ask: "Do you have difficulty driving or watching television or reading or doing any of your daily activities because of your eyesight?" If yes, then: Test each eye with Snellen chart while patient wears corrective lenses (if applicable)	Yes to question and inability to read > 20/40 on Snellen chart
Hearing	Use audioscope set at 40 dB; test hearing using 1000 and 2000 Hz	Inability to hear 1000 or 2000 Hz in both ears, or inability to hear frequencies in either ear
Leg mobility	Time the patient after asking: "Rise from the chair. Walk 20 feet briskly, turn, walk back to the chair, and sit down."	Unable to complete task in 15 sec

Problem	Screening Measure	Positive Screen
Urinary incontinence	Two parts: Ask: "In the past year, have you ever lost your urine and gotten wet?" If yes, then ask: "Have you lost urine on at least 6 separate days?"	Yes to both questions
Nutrition, weight loss	Two parts Ask: "Have you lost 10 lb over the past 6 months without trying to do so?" Weigh the patient	Yes to the question or weight < 100 lb
Memory	Three-item recall	Unable to recall all items after 1 min
Depression	Ask: "Do you often feel sad or depressed?"	Yes to the question
Physical disability	Six questions: "Are you able to..." "...do strenuous activities like fast walking or bicycling?" "...do heavy work around the house, like washing windows, walls, or floors?" "...go shopping for groceries or clothes?" "...get to places out of walking distance?" "...bathe, either a sponge bath, tub bath, or shower?" "...dress, like putting on a shirt, buttoning and zipping, or putting on shoes?"	No to any of the questions

Source: Reprinted from *Am J Med*, 100, Moore AA, Siu AL, Screening for common problems in ambulatory elderly: clinical confirmation of a screen instrument, 440, Copyright 1998, with permission from Excerpta Medica, Inc.

AUA SYMPTOM INDEX FOR BPH

Questions to be answered (circle 1 number on each line)	Not at all	Less than 1 time in 5	Less than half the time	About half the time	More than half the time	Almost always
1. Over the past month or so, how often have you had a sensation of not emptying your bladder completely after you finished urinating?	0	1	2	3	4	5
2. Over the past month or so, how often have you had to urinate again less than two hours after you finished urinating?	0	1	2	3	4	5
3. Over the past month or so, how often have you found you stopped and started again several times when you urinated?	0	1	2	3	4	5
4. Over the past month or so, how often have you found it difficult to postpone urination?	0	1	2	3	4	5
5. Over the past month or so, how often have you had a weak urinary stream?	0	1	2	3	4	5
6. Over the past month or so, how often have you had to push or strain to begin urination?	0	1	2	3	4	5
7. Over the last month, how many times did you most typically get up to urinate from the time you went to bed at night until the time you got up in the morning?	(none) 0	(1 time) 1	(2 times) 2	(3 times) 3	(4 times) 4	(5 or more times) 5

AUA Symptom Score = sum of questions 1–7 = _____. For interpretation, see p 133.

Source: Barry MJ, Fowler FJ Jr, O'Leary MP et al. The American Urological Association symptom index for benign prostatic hyperplasia. *J Urol.* 1992;148(5):1549–1557. Reprinted with permission.

OBRA REGULATIONS

US Health Care Financing Administration (in 2001 renamed Centers for Medicare and Medicaid Services) regulations regarding the use of certain medications in nursing homes are contained in the Omnibus Budget Reconciliation Act (OBRA) of 1987.

ANTIDEPRESSANT MEDICATIONS

Table 82. Recommended Maximum Doses of Antidepressants		
Drug	Usual Max Daily Dose (mg) for Age ≥ 65	Usual Max Daily Dose (mg)
Amitriptyline (*Elavil*)	150	300
Amoxapine (*Asendin*)	200	400
Desipramine (*Norpramin*)	150	300
Doxepin (*Adapin, Sinequan*)	150	300
Imipramine (*Tofranil*)	150	300
Maprotiline (*Ludiomil*)	150	300
Nortriptyline (*Aventyl, Pamelor*)	75	150
Protriptyline (*Vivactil*)	30	60
Trazodone (*Desyrel*)	300	600
Trimipramine (*Surmontil*)	150	300

ANTIPSYCHOTIC MEDICATIONS

Indications for appropriate use of antipsychotic medications are outlined in OBRA. In addition to psychotic disorders, these indications include specific nonpsychotic behavior associated with organic mental syndromes:
• Agitated psychotic symptoms (biting, kicking, scratching, assertive and belligerent behavior, sexual aggressiveness) that present a danger to themselves or others or interfere with family's and/or staff's ability to provide care (activities of daily living, or ADLs)
• Psychotic symptoms (hallucinations, delusions, paranoia)
• Continuous (24-h) crying out and screaming

Behavior less responsive to antipsychotic therapy includes:
• Repetitive, bothersome behavior (ie, pacing, wandering, repeated statements or words, calling out, fidgeting)
• Poor self-care
• Unsociability
• Indifference to surroundings
• Uncooperative behavior
• Restlessness
• Impaired memory
• Anxiety
• Depression
• Insomnia

If antipsychotic therapy is to be used for one or more of these symptoms only, then the use of antipsychotic agents is inappropriate. Because of their anticholinergic properties, antipsychotic agents may worsen these symptoms, especially symptoms of sedation and lethargy, as well as enhance "confusion."

Selection of an antipsychotic agent should be based on the side-effect profile since all antipsychotic agents are equally effective at equivalent doses. Coadministration of two or more antipsychotics does not have any pharmacologic basis or clinical advantage. Coadministration of two or more antipsychotic agents does not improve clinical response and increases the potential for side effects.

Once behavior control is obtained, assess patient to determine if precipitating event (stress from drugs, fluid or electrolyte changes, infection, changes in environment) has been resolved or patient has accommodated to the environment or situation. Determine whether the antipsychotic can be decreased in dose or tapered off completely by monitoring selected target symptoms for which the antipsychotic therapy was initiated. OBRA 1987 requires attempts at dose reduction within a 6-month period unless documented as to why this cannot be done. Identifying target symptoms is essential for adequate monitoring. Because of side effects, intermittent use (not prn) is preferable (ie, only when patient has behavior warranting use of these agents). For the recommended doses of antipsychotics, see **Table 83**.

Table 83. Recommended Maximum Doses of Antipsychotics			
Drug	Usual Max Daily Dose (mg) for Age ≥ 65	Usual Max Daily Dose (mg)	Daily Oral Dose (mg) for Residents with Organic Mental Syndromes
Acetophenazine (*Tindal*)	150	300	20
Chlorpromazine (*Thorazine*)	800	1600	75
Chlorprothixene (*Taractan*)	800	1600	75
Clozapine (*Clozaril*)	25	450	50
Fluphenazine (*Prolixin*)	20	40	4
Haloperidol (*Haldol*)	50	100	4
Loxapine (*Loxitane*)	125	250	10
Mesoridazine (*Serentil*)	250	500	25
Molindone (*Moban*)	112	225	10
Olanzapine (*Zyprexa*)	–	20	10
Quetiapine (*Seroquel*)	–	800	200
Perphenazine (*Trilafon*)	32	64	8
Promazine (*Sparine*)	50	500	150
Risperidone (*Risperdal*)	1	16	2
Thioridazine (*Mellaril*)	400	800	75
Thiothixene (*Navane*)	30	60	7
Trifluoperazine (*Stelazine*)	40	80	8
Triflupromazine (*Vesprin*)	100	20	–

ANXIOLYTIC MEDICATIONS

The use of anxiolytics is acceptable as long as other disease processes that could explain anxious behavior have been excluded. Daily use, at any dose, is for less than 4 continuous months, unless an attempt at dose reduction is unsuccessful. Proper indications include:

• Generalized anxiety disorder
• Organic mental syndrome (including dementia associated with agitation)
• Panic disorders
• Anxiety associated with other psychiatric disorder (eg, depression, adjustment disorder)

Table 84. Recommended Maximum Doses of Anxiolytics*		
Drug	Usual Daily Dose (mg) for Age ≥ 65	Usual Daily Dose (mg) for Age < 65
Alprazolam (*Xanax*)	2	4
Clorazepate (*Tranxene*)	30	60
Chlordiazepoxide (*Librium*)	40	100
Diazepam (*Valium*)	20	60
Halazepam (*Paxipam*)	80	160
Lorazepam (*Ativan*)	3	6
Meprobamate (*Miltown*)	600	1600
Oxazepam (*Serax*)	60	90
Prazepam (*Centrax*)	30	60

* HCFA-OBRA guidelines strongly urge clinicians not to use barbiturates, glutethimide, and ethchlorvynol because of their side effects, pharmacokinetics, and addiction potential in the elderly person. Also, HCFA discourages use of long-acting benzodiazepines in the elderly.

HYPNOTIC MEDICATIONS

Hypnotics are allowed for 10 continuous days of use. If three unsuccessful attempts at dose reduction occur, then it is clinically contraindicated to reduce.

Table 85. Recommended Maximum Doses of Hypnotics*		
Drug	Usual Max Single Dose (mg) for Age ≥ 65	Usual Max Single Dose (mg)
Alprazolam (*Xanax*)	0.25	1.5
Amobarbital (*Amytal*)	150	300
Butabarbital (*Butisol*)	100	200
Chloral hydrate (*Noctec*)	750	1500
Chloral hydrate (*various*)	500	1000
Diphenhydramine (*Benadryl*)	25	50
Ethchlorvynol (*Placidyl*)	500	1000
Flurazepam (*Dalmane*)	15	30
Glutethimide (*Doriden*)	500	1000
Halazepam (*Paxipam*)	20	40

Table 85. Recommended Maximum Doses of Hypnotics* (cont.)		
Drug	Usual Max Single Dose (mg) for Age ≥ 65	Usual Max Single Dose (mg)
Hydroxyzine (*Atarax*)	50	100
Lorazepam (*Ativan*)	1	2
Methyprylon (*Noludar*)	200	400
Oxazepam (*Serax*)	15	30
Phenobarbital (*Nembutal*)	100	200
Secobarbital (*Seconal*)	100	200
Temazepam (*Restoril*)	15	30
Triazolam (*Halcion*)	0.125	0.5

* HCFA-OBRA guidelines strongly urge clinicians not to use barbiturates, glutethimide, and ethchlorvynol because of their side effects, pharmacokinetics, and addiction potential in the elderly person. Also, HCFA discourages use of long-acting benzodiazepines in treating the elderly person.

HCFA CRITERIA: INAPPROPRIATE DRUG USE IN NURSING HOMES

On July 1, 1999, HCFA (the US Health Care Financing Administration, renamed in 2001 the Centers for Medicare and Medicaid Services) modified its regulations regarding medication use by nursing home residents who are 65 years of age or older. As part of their review, surveyors will determine if the resident is taking any medications considered to have a high potential ("high severity") for severe adverse drug reactions (ADRs) or medications with a high potential for less severe ("low severity") ADRs. Residents receiving any medications will be monitored for ADRs. If an ADR is identified, the rationale for the medication use must be justified and considered appropriate. If it is not, a deficiency will be cited.

Persons wishing additional information are advised to contact the American Society of Consultant Pharmacists (see p 230 for telephone number, Web site).

The medications specified in **Table 86** are considered "high severity" by HCFA and should be considered potentially inappropriate for use in treating elderly persons.

Table 86. Drugs Considered "High Severity" by HCFA	
Class or Drug	**Comments**
Amitriptyline (*Elavil*)	May be used for neurogenic pain if an evaluation of risk vs. benefit of the drug is documented, including consideration of alternative therapies
Chlorpropamide (*Diabinese*)	
Digoxin, in dosages > 0.125 mg/d	Unless an atrial arrhythmia is being treated; high severity is considered if started within the past month
Disopyramide (*Norpace*)	
GI antispasmodics (belladonna alkaloids, clidinium, dicyclomine, hyoscyamine, propantheline)	Use for short periods (not over 7 d) on an intermittent basis (not more frequently than q 3 mo) does not require review by the surveyor
Meperidine, oral	If started within past month
Methyldopa	If started within past month
Pentazocine	
Ticlopidine	Review by the surveyor is not necessary in individuals who receive it because they have had a previous stroke or have evidence of stroke precursors (ie, TIAs) and cannot tolerate aspirin

The drug-diagnosis combinations specified in **Table 87** are considered "high severity" by HCFA and should be considered potentially inappropriate for use in treating elderly persons.

178

Table 87. Diagnosis-Drug Combinations Considered "High Severity" by HCFA

Class or Drug	Diagnosis	Comments
Sedatives, hypnotics	COPD	Short-acting benzodiazepines are acceptable
NSAIDs	Active or recurrent gastritis, peptic ulcer disease, GERD	COX-2 inhibitors are not included on the list of NSAIDs
Metoclopramide	Seizures or epilepsy	
Aspirin, NSAIDs, dipyridamole, ticlopidine	Anticoagulation	
Anticholinergic drugs	BPH	
TCAs	Arrhythmias	If started within past month

The medications listed in **Table 88** are considered "low severity" by HCFA and should be considered as potentially inappropriate in treating elderly patients.

Table 88. Drugs Considered "Low Severity" by HCFA

Class or Drug	Comments
Antihistamines	That is, with anticholinergic properties
Cyclandelate	
Digoxin, in dosages > 0.125 mg/d	Unless an atrial arrhythmia is being treated; high severity is considered if started within the past month
Diphenhydramine	Review by a surveyor is not necessary if used for a short time (not over 7 d) on an intermittent basis (not more frequently than q 3 mo) for allergies
Dipyridamole	
Ergot mesylates (eg, *Hydergine*)	
Indomethacin	Short-term use (eg, 1 wk) is considered acceptable for treatment of gouty arthritis
Meperidine, oral	If therapy longer than 1 mo
Muscle relaxants (eg, carisoprodol, chlorzoxazone, cyclobenzaprine, dantrolene, metaxalone, methocarbarnol, orphenadrine)	Use for short periods (not over 7 d) on an intermittent basis (not more frequently than q 3 mo) does not require review

The drug-diagnosis combinations specified in **Table 89** are considered "low severity" by the HCFA and should be considered potentially inappropriate in all elderly patients.

Table 89 . Diagnosis-Drug Combinations Considered "Low Severity" by HCFA		
Class or Drug	**Diagnosis**	**Comments**
Corticosteroids	Diabetes mellitus	If started within past month
Potassium supplements or aspirin (> 325 mg/d)	Active or recurrent gastritis, peptic ulcer disease, or GERD	Use of potassium supplements to treat low potassium levels until they return to the normal range is permissible if prescriber determines that use of fresh fruits and vegetables or other dietary supplementation is not adequate or possible
Antipsychotics	Seizures or epilepsy	Treatment of acute psychosis for 72 h or less is permissible
Narcotic drugs, including propoxyphene	BPH	Review by the surveyor is not necessary if use is for short duration (7 d or less) on an intermittent basis (once q 3 mo) for symptoms of an acute, self-limiting condition
Bladder relaxants (flavoxate, oxybutynin, bethanechol)	BPH	Review by the surveyor is not necessary if use is for short duration (7 d or less) on an intermittent basis (once q 3 mo) for symptoms of an acute, self-limiting condition
Anticholinergic antihistamines, GI antispasmodics, anticholinergic antidepressants, and narcotic drugs (including propoxyphene)	Constipation	Constipation can be worsened Review by the surveyor is not necessary if use is for short duration (7 d or less) on an intermittent basis (once q 3 mo) for symptoms of an acute self-limiting condition
Antiparkinson medications	Constipation	Constipation can be worsened
Decongestants, theophylline, methylphenidate, SSRI antidepressants and desipramine, MAOIs, β-agonists	Insomnia	Insomnia can be worsened

INDEX

Page references followed by *t* and *f* indicate tables and figures, respectively.
Trade names are in *italics*.

Page references followed by *t* and *f* indicate tables and figures, respectively.
Trade names are in *italics*.

Page references followed by *t* and *f* indicate tables and figures, respectively.
Trade names are in *italics*.

Page references followed by *t* and *f* indicate tables and figures, respectively.
Trade names are in *italics*.

Page references followed by *t* and *f* indicate tables and figures, respectively.
Trade names are in *italics*.

189

Page references followed by *t* and *f* indicate tables and figures, respectively.
Trade names are in *italics*.

Page references followed by *t* and *f* indicate tables and figures, respectively.
Trade names are in *italics*.

Page references followed by *t* and *f* indicate tables and figures, respectively.
Trade names are in *italics*.

Page references followed by *t* and *f* indicate tables and figures, respectively.
Trade names are in *italics*.

Page references followed by *t* and *f* indicate tables and figures, respectively.
Trade names are in *italics*.

199

Page references followed by *t* and *f* indicate tables and figures, respectively.
Trade names are in *italics*.

201

Page references followed by t and f indicate tables and figures, respectively.
Trade names are in *italics*.

Page references followed by *t* and *f* indicate tables and figures, respectively.
Trade names are in *italics*.

Page references followed by *t* and *f* indicate tables and figures, respectively.
Trade names are in *italics*.

207

Page references followed by *t* and *f* indicate tables and figures, respectively.
Trade names are in *italics*.

Page references followed by *t* and *f* indicate tables and figures, respectively.
Trade names are in *italics*.

Page references followed by *t* and *f* indicate tables and figures, respectively.
Trade names are in *italics*.

Page references followed by *t* and *f* indicate tables and figures, respectively.
Trade names are in *italics*.

Page references followed by *t* and *f* indicate tables and figures, respectively.
Trade names are in *italics*.

217

Page references followed by *t* and *f* indicate tables and figures, respectively.
Trade names are in *italics*.

(continues)

219

Page references followed by *t* and *f* indicate tables and figures, respectively.
Trade names are in *italics*.

221

Page references followed by t and f indicate tables and figures, respectively. Trade names are in *italics*.

Page references followed by *t* and *f* indicate tables and figures, respectively.
Trade names are in *italics*.

ABOUT THE AMERICAN GERIATRICS SOCIETY

Founded in 1942, the American Geriatrics Society (AGS) is the leading clinical society devoted to the care of older adults. The AGS promotes high quality, comprehensive, and accessible care for America's older population, including those who are chronically ill and disabled. The organization provides leadership to health care professionals, policy makers, and the public by developing, implementing, and advocating programs in patient care, research, professional and public education, and public policy.

Its 6000 members include primary care physicians, geriatricians, geropsychiatrists, nurse practitioners, social workers, physician assistants, physical therapists, pharmacists, and others from the United States and around the world who are dedicated to improving the health, independence, and quality of life of the older population.

The AGS has long championed efforts to expand the national work force of clinicians with the specialized knowledge and skills to care for our aging population. Since the early 1990s, with funding from the John A. Hartford Foundation of New York City, the AGS has worked effectively to increase geriatrics expertise among subspecialists in internal medicine, practicing primary care physicians, and nonprimary care specialists.

In 1999, the AGS reached beyond its traditional role as a professional medical society and launched the **Foundation for Health in Aging (FHA)**. The FHA aims to build a bridge between the research/practice of geriatrics health care professionals and the public, and to advocate on behalf of older adults regarding issues of wellness and preventive care, self-responsibility and independence, and connections to family and community. For more information about FHA initiatives, please visit the Foundation website at www.healthinaging.org.

Current Major Publications and Programs of the AGS Include:
Journal of the American Geriatrics Society—rated in the top three of the ISI Science Citation Index for geriatrics and gerontology publications.

Geriatrics Review Syllabus: A Core Curriculum in Geriatric Medicine—the groundbreaking self-assessment, continuing education program for primary care providers and a premier source of clinically relevant information in geriatric medicine, now in its 5th edition.

Geriatrics At Your Fingertips—a comprehensive pocket-sized reference to clinical geriatrics that provides up-to-date, practical information on the evaluation and management of diseases and disorders most common to elderly people. Updated annually.

Annals of Long-Term Care: Clinical Care and Aging
This peer-reviewed journal presents the highest quality clinical reviews, analysis, and opinions that impact the present and future of long-term care, and is the premier source of information for professionals in the long-term care market.

Public Education Publications from the Foundation for Health in Aging—*Patient Education Forums* provide answers to commonly asked questions on a variety of geriatrics topics. *Eldercare at Home* is an extensive guide for families involved in providing care for older relatives who want to remain at home. Information on these and other public education programs is available on the Foundation website.

AGS Newsletter and AGS Website (www.americangeriatrics.org)—excellent sources of information on AGS activities and programs, noteworthy news, public policy issues, career opportunities in geriatrics, and much more.

Policy Position Statements and Clinical Practice Guidelines—In its Clinical Practice Guidelines series, the AGS, in collaboration with the British Geriatrics Society (BGS) and the American Academy of Orthopaedic Surgeons (AAOS), published *The Prevention of Falls in Older Persons* in the May 2001 issue of the *Journal of the American Geriatrics Society*. The AGS publishes position statements, papers, and guidelines to bring important issues in geriatrics education, research, clinical practice, and public policy to the attention of those working in the field, including policy makers, legislators, people in the health care industry, clinicians, and others.

The AGS Annual Scientific Meeting—the premier forum for the latest information on clinical geriatrics, research on aging and health problems of older adults, and innovative models in health care delivery as well as teaching in geriatrics.

The Geriatrics Recognition Award—awarded to recognize physicians and nurses who are committed to advancing their continuing education in geriatrics.

The AGS Awards Program—includes the following: the AGS Edward Henderson Award State-of-the-Art Lecture; AGS Clinician of the Year; AGS/Merck New Investigator Awards; Pfizer/AGS Postdoctoral Fellowship Awards; Dennis W. Jahnigen Memorial Award; the Nascher/Manning Award; the Otsuka/AGS Clinical Investigation Award; the Edward Henderson Student Award; and the AGS Student Research Award.

Special Projects in Professional Education/Outreach are funded by foundations and industry sponsors.

If you would like further information about the AGS, please contact us at:

The American Geriatrics Society
Empire State Building
350 5th Avenue, Suite 801
New York, NY 10118
www.americangeriatrics.org
or
Call the AGS
1-800-247-4779
or
E-mail
info.amger@americangeriatrics.org

IMPORTANT TELEPHONE NUMBERS AND WEB SITES

General Aging

AGS Foundation for Health in Aging	www.healthinaging.org	(212) 755-6810
American Association of Retired Persons	www.aarp.org	(800) 434-2277
American Geriatrics Society	www.americangeriatrics.org	(212) 308-1414
American Medical Directors Association	www.amda.com	(800) 876-2632
American Society of Consultant Pharmacists	www.ascp.com	(800) 355-2727
Assisted Living Federation of America	www.alfa.org	(703) 691-8100
Children of Aging Parents	www.caps4caregivers.org	(800) 227-7294
CDC National Prevention Information Network	www.cdcnpin.org	(800) 458-5231
Family Caregiver Alliance	www. caregiver.org	(800) 445-8106
Medicare Hotline	www.medicare.gov	(800) MEDICARE
National Adult Day Services Association	www.ncoa.org/nadsa	(202) 479-6682
National Council on the Aging	www.ncoa.org	(202) 479-1200
National Institute on Aging	www.nih.gov/nia	(800) 222-2225

Elder Abuse

National Center on Elder Abuse	www.elderabusecenter.org	(202) 898-2586

End-of-Life

National Hospice & Palliative Care Organization For hospice referral:	www.nhpco.org	(800) 658-8898

Specific Health Problems

Alzheimer's Association	www.alz.org	(800) 272-3900
Alzheimer's Disease Education & Referral Center	www.alzheimers.org	(800) 438-4380
American Academy of Ophthalmology	www.aao.org	(800) 222-3937
American Association for Geriatric Psychiatry	www.aagponline.org	(301) 654-7850
American Cancer Society, Inc.	www.cancer.org	(800) ACS-2345
American College of Obstetricians & Gynecologists	www.acog.com	(202) 638-5577
American Diabetes Association	www.diabetes.org	(800) DIABETES
American Foundation for the Blind	www.afb.org	(800) AFB-LINE
American Heart Association	www.americanheart.org	(800) AHA-USA1
American Lung Association	www.lungusa.org	(800) LUNG-USA
American Pain Society	www.ampainsoc.org	(847)-375-4715
American Parkinson Disease Association	www.apdaparkinson.com	(800) 223-2732
American Urological Association	www.auanet.org	(410) 727-1100
Arthritis Foundation	www.arthritis.org	(800) 283-7800

Better Hearing Institute	www.betterhearing.org	(800) EARWELL
Lighthouse International	www.lighthouse.org	(800) 829-0500
Meals On Wheels Association of America	www.projectmeal.org	(703) 548-5558
National Institute of Arthritis & Musculoskeletal & Skin Diseases	www.nih.gov/niams	(301) 496-8190
National Association for Continence	www.nafc.org	(800) BLADDER
National Diabetes Information Clearinghouse	www.niddk.nih.gov/health/diabetes/ndic.htm	(800) 860-8747
National Digestive Disease Information Clearinghouse	www.niddk.nih.gov/health/digest/nddic.htm	(800) 891-5389
National Eye Institute	www.nei.nih.gov	(301) 496-5248
National Heart, Lung & Blood Institute	www.nhlbi.nih.gov	(301) 592-8573
National Institute of Mental Health	www.nimh.nih.gov	(800) 421-4211
National Institute of Neurological Disorders & Stroke	www.ninds.nih.gov	(800) 352-9424
National Institute on Deafness & Other Communication Disorders	www.nidcd.nih.gov	TTY: (800) 241-1055; (800) 241-1044
National Kidney & Urologic Diseases Information Clearinghouse	www.niddk.nih.gov/health/kidney/nkudic.htm	(800) 891-5390
National Osteoporosis Foundation	www.nof.org	(800) 223-9994
National Parkinson Foundation	www.parkinson.org	(800) 327-4545
Self Help for Hard of Hearing People	www.shhh.org	TTY: (301) 657-2249; (301) 657-2248
Sexuality Information & Education Council of the US	www.siecus.org	(212) 819-9770
The Simon Foundation for Continence	www.simonfoundation.org	(800) 23-SIMON

GERIATRICS *At Your* FINGERTIPS
2002 Edition
From the American Geriatrics Society

A guide to the evaluation and management of the diseases and disorders that most commonly affect older persons.

Portable, Practical, Fully Indexed, and Up-to-Date!

Send completed order form with payment to:

Blackwell Publishing
c/o AIDC
PO Box 20
Williston, VT 05495-0020

For fast service
Call: 800-216-2522
Fax: 800-864-7626

Please send me _____ copies of Geriatrics At Your Fingertips, 2002 Edition @ $11.95 each

Subtotal   _____

Sales Tax (MA, VT and Canada)   _____

Shipping & Handling   _____
(No. Amer: $5.00 + $1.00 ea additional
Overseas: $8.00 + 1.00 ea additional)

TOTAL   _____

To order quantities of 25 or greater please contact our special sales department at 800-759-6102 X8341.

Method of Payment: _____ Check or money order payable to Blackwell

_____ MasterCard   _____VISA   _____AMEX

Card Number _____ Exp.Date _____

Signature _____

Shipping Instructions (must be complete)

Name: _____
Address: _____
City: _____State: _____ Zip: _____
Phone: _____
E-mail Address: _____

GAYF2002

Your request places you on the Blackwell e-alert electronic mailing list. You will be among the first in your discipline to find out about new releases, special offers and textbook announcements from Blackwell. After you receive your first e-alert, you have the option of canceling the service at any time. Prices subject to change without notice.